Ethnobotany: The Renaissance of Traditional Herbal Medicine

Ethnobotany: The Renaissance of Traditional Herbal Medicine

Ramesh Bhandari

CYBER TECH PUBLICATIONS
4264/3, Ansari Road, Daryaganj, New Delhi-110002 (India)
Ph.: 011-23244078, 011-43559448 Fax: 011-23280028
E-Mail: cyberpublicationsdelhi@yahoo.com
Website: www.cybertechpublications.com

ETHNOBOTANY: THE RENAISSANCE OF TRADITIONAL HERBAL MEDICINE

Ramesh Bhandari

First Edition 2010

Published by :

G.S. Rawat for **Cyber Tech Publications**
4264/3, Ansari Road, Daryaganj, New Delhi-110002 (India)
Ph.: 011-23244078, 011-43559448 Fax: 011-23280028
E-Mail: cyberpublicationsdelhi@yahoo.com
Website: www.cybertechpublications.com

Printed at: Asian Offset Printers, Delhi-53

Preface

These "useful" plants include many types of vegetation, including the herbaceous, flowering plants that come especially to mind when we think of herbs (such as parsley, basil, or thyme), as well as non-herbaceous trees and shrubs, vines, ferns, mosses, and other plant groups. The useful herbs include plants whose life cycles are annual (such as anise and basil), biennial (parsley, angelica, and clary sage), and perennial, including bay, lavender, lemon balm, thyme, yarrow, and many others. Specific herbs may be valued for their leaves (such as basil, bay, thyme), flowers (chamomile), seeds (dill, fennel), stems (angelica, chives), or underground parts (garlic, chicory). The notion of herbs as flavoring agents generally excludes those plants commonly known as vegetables, which are foods in and of themselves; that is, vegetables provide the substance, and herbs the seasoning. A related (and also imprecise) group of economic flora consists of the spice plants. These are generally understood to be plants, usually native to the tropics, that bear aromatic fruits, seeds, or woody barks, and that are used, although not solely, to season foods. (Cooking spices may also have medicinal, aromatic, or pesticidal properties.) Examples of culinary spices include cinnamon (consisting of the bark of a small evergreen tree native to Sri Lanka), black pepper (the unripe berries of a native Indonesian plant), and cloves (the dried flower buds of an evergreen tree from the Moluccas, known historically as the "Spice Islands.")

There is often confusion over which plants are herbs and which are spices. Herbs and spices have been used for many thousands of years. They provide a tangible link to ages past, when innumerable kinds of plants were an integral, daily part of home and community life. In Western societies prior to this century, people once turned to herbs to fulfill their physical and spiritual needs: to cure illness, season foods, and dye cloth; for their cosmetic properties and pleasing or repellent aromas; as well as for their magical or symbolic qualities. Although interest in particular herbs has waxed and waned over time and across cul-tures, we have witnessed a general decline in herbal popularity in the industrial era. Botanicals and other natural products have been eclipsed by purified or wholly synthetic drugs, food additives, chemical dyes and pesticides, and other manufactured products. This trend has been partially reversed in the late 20th Century, however, as shown by expanding herbal interest and activity from many quarters. This renewed focus consists, in part, of rediscovery and reevaluation of our pre- industrial herbal heritage, along with new interest in beneficial plants as renewable, biodegradable, or less-toxic resources, and greater interest in the cultural traditions of other groups.

In addition to their practical virtues, herbs are being newly appreciated for their beauty and versatility in the home garden. Many of our favorite ornamental garden flowers such as the rose, foxglove, and garden heliotrope are old-time herbs. Whether incorporated into the flower border, or herb or kitchen garden, herbs are being grown for their pleasing scents, interesting colors and textures, and their pest-deterrent properties. For our smaller living spaces, many herbs are suited to indoor culture and container gardens.

—Author

CONTENTS

1

Introduction

ETHNOBOTANY

Ethnobotany (*from "ethnology" - study of culture and "botany" - study of plants*) is the scientific study of the relationships that exist between people and plants. Ethnobotanists aim to reliably document, describe and explain complex relationships between cultures and (uses of) plants: focusing, primarily, on how plants are used, managed and perceived across human societies (e.g. as foods; as medicines; in divination; in cosmetics; in dyeing; as textiles; in construction; as tools; as currency; as clothing; in literature; in rituals; and in social life.)

History of Ethnobotany

Though the term "ethnobotany" was not coined until 1895 by the US botanist John William Harshberger, the history of the field begins long before that. In AD 77, the Greek surgeon Dioscorides published "*De Materia Medica*", which was a catalog of about 600 plants in the Mediterranean. It also included information on how the Greeks used the plants, especially for medicinal purposes. This illustrated herbal contained information on how and when each plant was gathered, whether or not it was poisonous, its actual use, and whether or not it was edible (it even provided recipes). Dioscorides stressed the economic potential of plants. For generations, scholars learned from this herbal, but did not actually venture into the field until after the Middle Ages.

In 1542 Leonhart Fuchs, a Renaissance artist, led the way back into the field. His "*De Historia Stirpium*" cataloged 400 plants native to Germany and Austria.

John Ray (1686-1704) provided the first definition of "species" in his "*Historia Plantarum*": a species is a set of individuals who give rise through reproduction to new individuals similar to themselves.

In 1753 Carl Linnaeus wrote "*Species Plantarum*", which included information on about 5,900 plants. Linnaeus is famous for inventing the binomial method of nomenclature, in which all species get a two part name (genus, species). The 19th century saw the peak of botanical exploration. Alexander von Humboldt collected data from the new world, and the James Cook's voyages brought back collections and information on plants from the South Pacific. At this time major botanical gardens were started, for instance the Royal Botanic Gardens, Kew. Edward Palmer collected artifacts and botanical specimens from peoples in the North American West (Great Basin) and Mexico from the 1860s to the 1890s.

Once enough data existed, the field of "aboriginal botany" was founded. Aboriginal botany is the study of all forms of the vegetable world which aboriginal peoples use for food, medicine, textiles, ornaments, etc. The first individual to study the emic perspective of the plant world was a German physician working in Sarajevo at the end of 19th Century: Leopold Glueck. His published work on traditional medical uses of plants done by rural people in Bosnia (1896) has to be considered the first modern ethnobotanical work.

The term "ethnobotany" was first used by a botanist named John W. Harshberger in 1895 while he was teaching at the University of Pennsylvania. Although the term was not used until 1895, practical interests in ethnobotany go back to the beginning of civilization when people relied on plants as a way of survival.

Other scholars analysed uses of plants under an indigenous/ local perspective in the 20th century: e.g. Matilda Coxe Stevenson, Zuni plants (1915); Frank Cushing, Zuni foods (1920); Keewaydinoquay Peschel, Anishinaabe fungi (1998), and the team approach of Wilfred Robbins, JP Harrington, and Barbara Freire-Marreco, Tewa pueblo plants (1916).

In the beginning, ethonobotanical specimens and studies were not very reliable and sometimes not helpful. This is because the botanists and the anthropologists did not come together on their work. The botanists focused on identifying species and how the plants were used instead of including how plants fit into people's lives. On the other hand, anthropologists were interested in the cultural role of plants and not the scientific aspect. Therefore, early ethnobotanical data does not really include both sides. In the early twentieth century, botanists and anthropologists finally collaborated and the collection of reliable, detailed data began.

Modern Ethnobotany

Beginning in the 20th century, the field of ethnobotany experienced a shift from the raw compilation of data to a greater methodological and conceptual reorientation. This is also the beginning of academic ethnobotany. The founding father of this discipline is Richard Evans Schultes. Today the field of ethnobotany requires a variety of skills: botanical training for the identification and preservation of plant specimens; anthropological training to understand the cultural concepts around the perception of plants; linguistic training, at least enough to transcribe local terms and understand native morphology, syntax, and semantics.

Considerable information on the traditional uses of plants is still intact with the tribals. But the native healers are often reluctant to accurately share their knowledge to outsiders. Schultes actually apprenticed himself to an Amazonian shaman, which involves a long term commitment and genuine relationship. In *Wind in the Blood: Mayan Healing & Chinese Medicine* by Garcia et al. the visiting acupuncturists were able to access levels of Mayan medicine that anthropologists could not because they had something to share in exchange. Cherokee medicine priest David Winston describes how his uncle would invent nonsense to satisfy visiting anthropologists.

2

Use of Herbal Medicine Against Helminths in Livestock

Helminths are recognized as a major constraint to livestock production throughout the tropics and elsewhere (Waller, 1987; Ibrahim *et al.*, 1984). Imported manufactured anthelmintics have long been considered the only effective way of controlling parasitic infection. However, as these are very expensive and often unavailable to farmers in rural areas, livestock producers have continued to use indigenous plants as dewormers, drawing upon centuries of knowledge of herbal medicine. Furthermore, some serious disadvantages of using manufactured drugs have become evident in the western world, such as drug resistance, food residues and environmental pollution. A general stagnation in the development of conventional medicine has led to an increased need for research into alternative therapeutic agents for the treatment and control of helminth infections. Knowledge about medicinal plants is not new to the western world; rather, it has been forgotten - 25 percent of all prescriptions dispensed in public pharmacies in the United States in 1973 contained drugs extracted from higher plants (Farnsworth and Morris, 1976).

Similarly, some plants have been listed as anthelmintics in the British Veterinary Codex, at least until 1965. Extensive medicinal knowledge is to be found through research on the traditional use of herbal medicine, since an estimated 80 percent of the populations of developing countries depend on traditional medicines for primary health care (WHO, cited by Plotkin, 1992). The same figure seems to hold for livestock and ethnoveterinary care (McCorkle *et al.*, 1996). It is considered that further research into this area will benefit both developed and less developed countries.

This review presents some examples of herbal medicine used against helminths in livestock, and outlines potentials and limitations in the use of ethnomedicine, or ethnobotanical medicine - the utilization by humans of plants as medicines (Farnsworth, 1994). "Traditional" refers to the sum total of all non-mainstream medical practices, usually excluding so-called "western" medicine (Farnsworth, 1994). "Ethnoveterinary medicine" is defined as being the study of folk beliefs, knowledge, skills, methods and practices on the part of practitioners concerned with the health care of animals (McCorkle, 1989).

USE OF TRADITIONAL HERBAL MEDICINE

There is an increased awareness among medical and scientific communities that the importance of medicinal plant studies goes beyond mere anthropological curiosity. Plant anthelmintics have been in the forefront of this growing awareness (Hammond, Fielding and Bishop, 1997). A reason for this could be that they fall into the category of readily applicable elements of ethnoveterinary medicine in livestock development (McCorkle and Mathias-Mundy, 1992). Studying herbal medicine can serve to validate and enhance existing local uses and can give clues to remedies with further potential. There are, however, other reasons for continuing interest and research.

First of all, locally produced plant anthelmintics are much cheaper than imported drugs. One striking example is a herbal wound powder in Sri Lanka, found to be as effective as an imported powder, which cost 80 to 90 percent less than the western equivalent (Anjaria, 1986). Logically, peasant farmers choose not to buy the western drugs and this may make availability a problem in rural areas, as a result of lower demand. Safe, efficacious and high-quality anthelmintic products are a normal requirement in many countries. Unfortunately, they are not always available. A recent investigation found plausible evidence of direct fraud with commercially available products. This led Monteiro *et al.* (1997) to compare the actual content of active drugs with the contents claimed on the labels of nine anthelmintic products sold in Kenya. They found that the actual levamisole concentration varied from 0 to 114 percent and that the concentration in different batches of the same product varied from 0 to 85 percent.

These deviations could be owing either to incorrect storage or to deliberate fraud, such as dilution. The effect of a product with no active drug is the continued suffering of the animal and lower production. Use of anthelmintic products with inadequate amounts of the active ingredient will, in turn, encourage the development of anthelmintic resistance, since sub-optimal dosing selects for chemoresistant populations (Martin, 1990) and overdosing can result in residual amounts in the faeces, which may influence resistance further. Illiteracy or unfamiliarity with imported anthelmintics, resulting in incorrect usage, is also a problem leading to the same consequences.

These constraints in the use of synthetic western anthelmintics in less developed countries underline the advantages of herbal remedies as an alternative treatment. They are cheaper and more reliable, they are known by the users and their supply is more sustainable. As they have undergone many years of clinical trials, most of them do not contain acutely toxic plants and do not produce serious unanticipated side-effects. Since they do not contain substances such as fixatives, preservatives or hormones, they are presumably more biodegradable and lead to less bioaccumulation in patients' bodies and the environment (McCorkle, 1995). Furthermore, it has been suggested that the diversity of herbal anthelmintics has precluded the occurrence of resistance despite many years of use, as discussed above (Hammond, Fielding and Bishop, 1997).

Greater and more organized use of herbal medicine as a whole also supports the Convention on Biological Diversity, which at the June 1992 United Nations Conference on Environment and

Development in Rio de Janeiro was signed by 154 countries (excluding the United States) and initiated in December 1993, after final ratification by 30 countries (Government of Denmark, 1996). The Convention aims at a commitment to cooperation between the contracting countries with regard to the conservation and sustainable use of the diversity of animals, plants and other living organisms and their habitats. Wider use of traditional herbal medicine can help fulfil these aims through the organized use of medicinal plants. Furthermore, the Convention seeks a reasonable division of the profit from the use of genetic resources.

A country thus has a sovereign right over its resources (Government of Denmark, 1996, article 3) and is thereby assured of a monetary share in the possible marketing of a product from these natural resources. Organized cultivation of medicinal herbs and the creation of local trade and industry based on the herbal products can bring more jobs, income and status to rural inhabitants (McCorkle, 1995). Maintaining biodiversity in turn maintains the cultural diversity that is reflected in the people who administer the biodiverse habitats (Hyndman, 1994).

These goals can be accomplished through ethnoveterinary research, development and extension (ERD&E / ER&D), which can be defined as "the holistic, interdisciplinary study of local knowledge and its associated skills, practices, beliefs, practitioners and social structures pertaining to the health care and healthful husbandry of food-, work- and other income-producing animals, always with an eye to practical development applications within livestock production and livelihood systems, and with the ultimate goal of increasing human well-being via increased benefits from stock raising" (McCorkle, 1995). The appreciation of traditional herbal medicine promoted by ER&D may lead to increased recognition of indigenous knowledge - the local knowledge unique to a given culture or society (Warren, 1995) - as a potential scientific resource. This may be regarded as one of the most important aspects of the re-emergence of herbal medicine.

PROBLEMS WITH THE USE OF TRADITIONAL HERBAL MEDICINE

The case of ethnomedicine, human and veterinary, is not all straightforward. Because it is a very new area of academic study, many scientists and veterinarians still consider it pure superstition without a place in reality, the domain of "quacks" (Mesfin and Obsa, 1994). The main reason for this scepticism is basically a natural doubt about all that is alien and different, which all traditional methods must be to the western eye. Ethnomedicine does not follow western paradigms of scientific proof of efficacy, which might be one of the main arguments against the use of traditional medicine today (Sofowora, 1982). On the other hand, this may be one of the constraints that is easiest to reverse in the future, using organized investigative methods for scientific evaluation.

Among the limitations of ethnoveterinary medicine, Mathias-Mundy and McCorkle (1989) mention "the inconvenience of preparing or using some remedies, the seasonal availability of certain plants, the scarcity of treatments against infectious epidemic diseases, the ineffectiveness of some treatments, the existence of harmful practices and the often inadequate ethno-diagnoses".

The inconvenience of using some traditional remedies lies with the problems of collecting, preparing and administering the ingredients, which in some cases can be very time-consuming. Each constituent has to be found in special habitats and some ingredients might be seasonal. However, stock owners also have to go far to get imported medicine, which is currently the case in many rural areas in developing countries. The problem of time-consuming collection of some medicinal plants could be solved by organizing the most important of them into cultivation schemes. Seasonal availability, however, could not be overcome in this way, but developing proper storage techniques might be a solution.

Inadequate ethnodiagnosis is probably the weakest aspect of traditional health care practice, owing to a lack of pathophysiological understanding (Schillhorn van Veen, 1997). The understanding of disease causality is rarely developed, and hence treatment and prevention can be inappropriate. Lack of sophisticated modern diagnostic technology for proper diagnosing is also a problem, even when the cause of disease is understood. For instance, helminths might only be recognized when they are of a size that makes them visible in faeces. Recognition of parasite eggs and small worms and differentiation between species is in some cases difficult without even a microscope. Differential diagnosis of helminth diseases from other conditions can also be a problem, since gross clinical signs such as weight loss, diarrhoea and anaemia could be caused by many ailments other than helminthosis.

Poor diagnosis leads to some of the other constraints mentioned in the use of traditional medicine. Ineffectiveness of some treatments follows partly from poor diagnosis, leading to the application of inappropriate treatments. For instance, some plants only have a laxative effect and may expel only adult worms or parts of worms (Hammond, Fielding and Bishop, 1997). Furthermore, inadequate diagnosis or a lack of understanding of the disease can also lead to harmful prescriptions. In the case of a bacterial disease such as anthrax, which can be transmitted from animals to humans, the danger is not always known and the disease may be spread accidentally by the consumption of contaminated meat (Bizimana, 1994). Another human example (Bourke and Petana, 1994) was an African miner who complained of abdominal pain and nausea. He consulted a native medicine man, who advised that a mixture should be prepared from the segments of the worm (*Taenia solium*) the miner had brought with him. He drank the mixture and was subsequently hospitalized with epilepsy and muscular pain. X-rays of his body showed multiple cystercerci in the musculature. The liquid had probably contained thousands of ova, which resulted in this condition with cystercerci in the musculature and brain tissue. It shortly thereafter caused his death.

Stories such as these understandably support the view of ethnomedicine as the domain of "quacks", not always without reason. Many traditional healers would never admit to a lack of knowledge. In some cases they would just order a remedy with no effects, or in the worst cases even harmful ones, in order to keep their reputation (Hammond, Fielding and Bishop, 1997) or simply to make money. However, the above example of the wrong treatment most probably does not originate from ill intentions or motives, but simply from a lack of understanding.

Western science normally maintains a clear division between medicine and religion, so magico-religious practices are another cause of suspicion. In human ethnomedicine, as well as in ethnoveterinary medicine, magic and religion are integral parts of the whole (McCorkle, 1986) although Nwude and Ibrahim (1980) find the mystic rites that surround human traditional medicine virtually non-existent.

Supernatural practices vary from simple recitations or incantations to complex ceremonies (Mathias-Mundy and McCorkle, 1989). Although such actions might have a psychosomatic effect in humans, their value in animals is uncertain. However, some factual knowledge with practical value may be hidden in magico-religious expressions. In ethnopharmacology, some remedies that were used for magic or symbolic purposes have been proved effective scientifically (McCorkle and Mathias-Mundy, 1992). Studying natural practices without the supernatural is hence "scientifically indefensible" (McCorkle and Mathias-Mundy, 1992).

How to Go Forward?

To use the words of Plotkin (1992), veterinary and human ethnomedicine stand at a crossroads. The decline and possible disappearance of all traditional practices lie in one direction, as traditional cultures come into contact with the western world. In the other far more desirable direction lie validation and improvement of ethnomedical knowledge.

The collection and testing of natural products is one of two ways to discover pharmaceuticals; the other is laboratory synthesis (Soejarto, 1996). Different approaches can be used to collect products such as plants with anthelmintic properties.

The biodiversity-based approach, also called the random collection and screening approach, involves the screening of a large set of diverse plant samples for one or more biological activities (Soejarto, 1996). The reservoir for discovery is almost inexhaustible, as it contains all plant species. However, this undoubtedly makes it the more expensive approach, considering the relatively low chances of discovery. A second approach is field observations for signs of interaction between organisms. This is based on the idea that plant secondary metabolites are a defence for the plant, acting against potential predators or pathogens such as viruses, bacteria, nematodes and others (Whitfield, 1995). A third approach arises from this, namely the selection of plants based on chemotaxonomy, since plant secondary metabolites are often species- or family-specific in their taxonomic distribution (Whitfield, 1995).

Finally, the ethnobotanical approach and investigation of self-medicating behaviour in animals (Huffman, 1997) offer opportunities for the discovery of medicinal plants. The ethnobotanical approach assumes that the indigenous use of plants can give hints about their biological activities (Cox and Balick, 1994).

A comparison with human ethnomedicine is important for the discovery of veterinary plant anthelmintics, because in many cultures healers of human diseases treat corresponding animal disorders with the same herbs, drugs, methods, etc. (Mathias-Mundy and McCorkle, 1989; Nwude and Ibrahim, 1980).

The follow-up investigation of the ethnomedical uses of plants is widely accepted as the most productive plant surveying method, since 74 percent of all plant-derived drugs in clinical use worldwide have been discovered in this way (Farnsworth *et al.*, 1985). Information on plants used medically can be obtained through literature search and analysis, and through field inquiries, although this makes it a very slow process.

This is one of the limitations to this approach, and at the same time what constitutes its urgency. Rapid social and agricultural changes are taking place in many rural communities and therefore it is necessary to collect information on traditional patterns of use before these are disrupted. Many healers possessing information are elderly and lack successors and, as they die, their knowledge dies with them (Cox and Balick, 1994).

However, reliance on healers' information might not be so important when collecting information on ethnoveterinary practices, because healers of human ailments keep their knowledge secret, while ethnoveterinary information circulates freely. Herders often possess knowledge of gross pathology through slaughtering, while human healers base their diagnoses solely on symptoms (Mathias-Mundy and McCorkle, 1989).

Another constraint to the ethnobotanical approach is the limitation of indigenous plant use to certain recognized disorders which do not fully correspond to the diseases western medicine concentrates on. Indigenous plant remedies are more focused on gastro-intestinal complaints, inflammation, dermatological ailments and obstetric disorders (Cox and Balick, 1994), which in the case of discovering anthelmintic herbs must be considered significant.

The most promising plants should be scientifically validated through systematic experiments, using indicator helminths in laboratory animals and toxicity studies and, if these are positive, screening in domestic animals (Hammond, 1997). In this way two plants, *Embelia schimperi* and *Carica papaya*, were found by the Danish Centre for Experimental Parasitology to be promising anthelmintic candidates (Bøgh, Andreassen and Lemmich, 1996; Satrija *et al.*, 1994, 1995). For further examples see the Table. To ensure benefit to the inhabitants, the plants should, as far as possible, be cultivated and packaged locally and commercially marketed.

CONCLUSION

The advantages of studying local knowledge of herbal medicine are numerous and most of them have already been outlined here. To sum up, it is important, in both a socio-economic and a scientific perspective, to draw upon the rich store of ethnomedicinal knowledge. Herbal medicine is still used by the majority of humans on earth, mainly among populations in less developed countries. To these people, herbal medicines offer cheaper, more sustainable, available, reliable and familiar alternatives to imported synthetic drugs. Furthermore, when put into production locally, they can reinforce the income and status of local inhabitants.

For both developed and less developed countries, the recognition and development of herbal medicine offers treatment methods that are more environmentally benign, since they tend to be less toxic, produce fewer unanticipated side-effects, are more biodegradable, accumulate no drug residues in meat or faeces and apparently do not trigger anthelmintic chemoresistance.

However, there are problems connected with the use of herbal medicine, the largest being the lack of scientific evaluation. Such evaluation is the most important step once information about indigenous uses of medicinal plants has been collected. The most effective approach to obtaining such knowledge is the ethnobotanical approach, which assumes that indigenous uses of plants indicate the presence of biologically active constituents in the plants.

This is a slow but very urgent process, as young people desert the traditional knowledge and lifestyles of their elders, leading to the possible disappearance of this knowledge. Comparison with human ethnomedicine is also important when looking for plants against ailments of livestock, since healers often use the same medications for similar animal diseases.

Finally, ER&D offers a way to obtain ethnoveterinary practices as it seeks sustainable development through appreciating and building upon local knowledge of veterinary and husbandry practices. In this way, herbal medicine may very well become a pioneer in turning local knowledge into global knowledge, through the recognition of local knowledge as an indispensable source of sustainable development for both people and the environment all over the world. This of course does not mean that traditional medicine should take over western medicine, but rather that we may benefit from a harmonious balance of both.

Plants reported to be traditionally used as anthelmintics

Plant	Part used	Active constituent	Indication cited or activity	Animal species
Acacia albida	Seeds		Worm infestation	Sheep, goat
Agrimonia eupatori			Anthelmintic	Humans
Alangium lamarckii	Root-bark		Ascarids	Poultry
Albizia anthelmintica	Bark RootBark		Anthelmintic	Cattle, goat,
			Fasciolosis,	sheep Cattle, goat,
			lungworms	sheep, camel
Albizia coriavera	BarkBulb		Fasciolosis,	Cattle, goat,
Allium sativum			lungworms	sheep Cattle, goat,
			Roundworms	sheep
Aloe barteri	Leaves	Anthraquin one	Nippostrongyllus braziliensis	Rat
Ananas comosus	Fruit		Ascaridia galli	Chicken
Annona cherimolia		Acetogenins	Nippostroongylus	Rat
A. muricata braziliensis				
Molinema dessetae				
A. senegalensis	Leaf, bark, root	Anthraquinone	Nippostrongyllus braziliensis	Rat

Anogeissus leiocarpus	Bark, seed	Anthraquinone	Nippostrongyllus braziliensis	Rat
Areca catechu	Nut	Arecolin, other alkaloids	Taenicidal	Cattle, goat, dog
Artemisia maritima		Santonin, Artemisin	Neoascaris vitulorum	Buffalo calves
Bixa orellana	Seeds		Ascaridia galli, Ascaris suum	Chicken Pig
Boswellia dalzelii	Bark		Anthelmintic	Sheep, goat
Butea frondosa			Oxyurids	Mice
	Seeds		Ascaridia galli	In vitro
Caesalpina crista	Seeds		Toxocara vitulorum Ascaridia galli	Buffalo calves Chicken
Callindra portoricensis	Root		Toxocara canis	Dog
Carica papaya	Latex from fruit		Ascaridia galli Ascaris suum Heligmosomoides polygyrus	Chicken Pig Mice
Carissa edulis	>Root		Roundworms	Cattle, goat, sheep
Cassia alata	Seeds		Ascaridia galli	Chicken
Cassia occidentalis	Leaf	Anthraquinone	Nippostrongylus braziliensis	Rat

Cassia spectalis	Root		Roundworms	Cattle, goat, sheep
Chrysanthemum spp.		Pyrethrin	Ascaridia lineata	Chicken
Chrysophyllum cainito	Stem		Haemonchus contortus	Cattle
Cissampelos mucromata	Root		Anthelmintic	
Clitorea ternatea	Seeds		Ascaridia galli	Chicken
Combretum mucronatum	Root		Guinea worm	Humans
Croton macrostachys	Leaves		Anthelmintic	
Diospyros mespilliformis	>Bark		Anthelmintic	
Diospyros mollis		Diospyrol	Necator americanus	Golden hamster Nematodirus dubius, Hymenolepis nana Mice
Diospyrus scabra	Seeds		Fasciolosis, lungworms	Cattle, goat, sheep, camel
Dodonea viscosa	Leaves		Intestinal worms	
Embelia kilimandschiraca	Root		Anthelmintic	
Embelia Schimperi	Seed, root		Anthelmintic	
	Fruit	Embelin	Hymenolepis diminuta	Rat

Erythrina senegalensis	Bark		Fasciolosis	Ruminants
Evodia rutaecarpa		Atanin	Ascarid nematodes	Pig (in vitro),
	L4 of . Ostertagia circ		Sheep (in vitro)	
Hagenia abyssainica	Fruit		Roundworms	Cattle, goat, sheep
Lansium domesticum	Seeds		Ascaridia galli	Chicken, Pig, Goat
			Ascaris suun Haemonchus contortus	
Lantana trifolia	Fruit		Fasciolosis, lungworms	Cattle, goat, sheep
Lawsonia inermis	Leaf		Fasciolosis	Sheep, goat
Leucaena leucocephala	Seeds		Ascaridia galli	Chicken, Pig, Goat
			Ascaris suum Haemonchus contortus	
Mangifera indica	Seeds		Ascaridia galli •	Chicken
Mallotus philippinensis			Gastro-intestinal cestodes	Beetal goat
Melia azederach	Fruit		Ascaridia galli	Chicken
			Haemonchus, Tricho- strongylus, Trichuris, Chabertia spp.	Goat

Mimosa pudica	Stem		Haemonchus contortus	
Mitragyna stipulosa	Root		Guinea worm	Humans
Momordica charantia	Stem		Ascaris suum	Pig, Chicken
			Ascaridia galli	
			Haemonchus contortus	Goat
Moringa oleifera	Seeds		Ascaridia galli	Chicken, Pig, Goat
			Ascaris suum	
			Haemonchus contortus	
Myrsine africana	Leaf		Roundworms	Cattle, goat, sheep, donkey, camel
Peganum harmala	Seeds	Tetra-hydroharmin	Mixed gastrointestinal infection	Goat
			Cestiod infection	Sheep
Quisqualis indica	Stem		Ascaris suum,	Pig
			Ascaridia galli	Chicken
			Haemonchus contortus	Goat

Rapanea melanoploeos	Seeds		Roundworms	Cattle, goat, sheep
Rhamnus principides	Leaves		Anthelmintic	Minja (1989)
Rhus vulgaris	Root		Roundworms	Cattle, goat, sheep
Senecio lyratiparitus	Leaves		Anthelmintic	.
Solanum nodiflorum	Fruit		Worm infestation	
Tamarindus indica	Root		Roundworms	Cattle, goat, sheep
Terminalia avicennoides	Leaf, root		Anthraquinone	Nipposrongylus braziliensis
Tiinospora rumphii	Stem		Haemonchus contortus	Goat
Tribulus terestris	Plant		Ascaridia galli	Poultry
Trichilia emetica	Bark		Fasciolosis, lungworms	Cattle, goat, sheep, camel
Uvaria hookeri	Root-bark	Acetogenins	Haemonchus contortus	
U. narum				
Vernonia anthelmintica			Oxyurids	Mice

3

Medicinal Plants in an Urban Environment

Varanasi is one of the oldest continuously inhabited cities of the world, and one of the most important Hindu pilgrimage sites. Despite this importance, very little information exits on the cities flora in general, and medicinal species found within its limit in particular. Traditional medicine plays a large role in Indian society. The presented study attempted to investigate if traditional plant use and availability of important common medicinal plants are maintained in urban environments. The paper presents information on the traditional uses of seventy-two plant species collected form the campus of Banares Hindu University, Varanasi, Uttar Pradesh, and highlights the uses of these plants by the local inhabitants.

BACKGROUND

Traditional medicine based on herbal remedies has always played a key role in the health systems of many countries. In India the native people are exploiting a variety of herbals for effective curing of various ailments. The plant parts used, preparation, and administration of drugs vary from one place to other. However, the knowledge of herbal medicines is gradually perishing, although some of the traditional herbal men are still practicing the art of herbal healing effectively. These plants are frequently used by the local inhabitants of the area for treatment of various diseases. Ethno-medicinal studies have offered immense scope and opportunities for the development of new drugs. Some modern drugs have been deducted from folklore and traditional medicines. Living close to nature, traditional societies have acquired unique knowledge about the use of wild flora and fauna, most of which are unknown to the people who live away from such natural ecosystem as forests. After years of observations and analysis, trials, error, experimentation or even use of intuitive methods the innovative member of human communities have selected/identified useful and harmful members of the flora and fauna.

Such knowledge and practices/experience were subjected to further modification or enriched with new knowledge of practice by succeeding generations and become a part of the tradition, culture, art, belief, folklore and knowledge base of these traditional communities. The traditional knowledge, skill and practices thus developed are freely exchanged cared for and nourished as a common property of the communities.

The value and importance of traditional knowledge are now being increasingly acknowledge all over the world. The pharmaceutical industry continues to investigate and confirm the efficacy of many medicines and toxins used by traditional communities.

The forests have been the source of invaluable medicinal plants since the time man realized the preventive and curative properties of plants and started using them for human heath care. The old traditional Indian Systems of Medicine (ISM), is one of the most ancient medicine practices known to the world, and derives maximum formulations from plants and plant extracts that exist in the forests. About 400 plants are used in regular production of Ayurvedic, Unani, Siddha and tribal medicine. About 75% are from tropical and 25% from temperate forests. 30% of preparations are derived from roots, 14% bark, 16% whole plants, 5% flowers, 10% fruits, 6% leaves, 7% seeds, 3% wood, 4% rhizomes 6% stems and only less than 20% of the species used are cultivated.

Forest degradation processes adversely affect the resource base of medicinal plants. The rural poor, whose dependence on these products is very heavy, are the worst sufferers. The problems are compounded by market-demand driven harvesting without any concern for representation and conservation. In the process essential regenerative components of a plant like roots, tubers, fruits, seeds flowers and bark are indiscriminately collected, leading to degradation and depletion and even extinction of particular species. Due to this ruthless exploitation, many important medicinal plants species are becoming rare and some of them are critically endangered. It is estimated that 10% of all plant species are currently endangered in India.

The study was performed in and around the area of Banaras Hindu University campus. Varanasi is one of the oldest continuously inhabited cities of the world, and one of the most important Hindu pilgrimage sites. Despite this importance, very little information exits on the cities flora in general, and medicinal species found within its limit in particular.

The city lies at latitudes 82°50' E to 83°03' E and longitude 25°10' N to 25°25' N at an altitude of approximately 79.1 m above the sea level, with fairly level topography. Varanasi has a humid subtropical climate with high variation between summer and winter temperatures. Summers are long, from early April till October, with the monsoon season in between. Cold waves from the Himalayan region dip temperatures across the city in the winter from December to February. The average temperature is 32°C-46°C in summer; 5°C-15°C in the winter. The average annual rainfall is 1110 mm. Fog is common in winter while hot dry winds called loo blow in summer. Soils are generally old alluvial deposits of the middle Gangetic plain.

Methods

A plant inventory was conducted in and around the campus of Banaras Hindu University. All plants were collected, identified, and vouchers were stored at the herbarium of the Department of Dravya Guna, Faculty of Ayurved, Institute of Medical Science, Banares Hindu University, under the first author's collector series. The field survey covered different seasons. The survey was started in rainy seasons (August) and collections were repeated every month for two years. Seasonal variations and frequency of plant occurrence were noted.

Ethnomedicinal uses of the plants were first extracted from the relevant literature available in the library of the university. The ethnomedicinal uses mentioned in literature were then cross checked through interviews with local inhabitants in the villages and urban areas surrounding the university campus and visits to the local Kavirag and Vaidyas who act as are plant collectors and local healers. The interviews were conducted randomly after obtaining prior informed consent of the participants. Only those ethnomedicinal uses agreed upon by a majority of informants were retained. The study did not involve interviews with tribal ethnic groups, and the dosages, specific formulations and mode of administration were recorded, but retained as intellectual property of the informants.

During the field visit the survey of data collection was made in different places i.e. waste lands, bare lands, play ground, road side, agricultural farms and near other localities. The collected samples of plants were brought to the department for identification.

Data on medicinal/ethnomedicinal uses of plants are presented in additional file in the following sequences: serial number, botanical name, family, vernacular name, part used, life form and ethnomedicinal uses.

Results and Discussion

India has a tradition of codified healthcare systems: Ayurveda, Unani and Siddha, functions mainly through (1) folk stream and (2) classical stream. The former, is based on oral traditions, practiced by villagers and the tribal communities while the later comprises the codified systems supported by theoretical knowledge, experimental and philosophical explanations provided by many learned physicians and surgeons of earlier time like Charak, Sushruta, Galen, Rhazes, Avicenna, and others. The preventive, corrective and curative approaches of health is the basic strength of the Indian Systems of Medicine (ISM), which are mostly plant based and comprise over

8000 medicinal and aromatic plants species. In India, about 1.5 million practitioners of ISM use around 25000 effective plant based formulations. According to the all Indian co-ordinate project sponsored by the Ministry of Environment of Forests, New Delhi, 40% of the 16,000 recorded flowering plants in India have ethno-medicinal value, whereas, only 10% of these are used in drug and pharmaceutical industries. The intrinsic importance of these medicinal plants can very well prove as a potential source of new drugs.

No survey of naturally growing medicinal plants of the present study area has been reported till date. Duthie's work on the flora of upper Gangetic plain and of the adjacent Siwalik and Sub-Himalayan tracts included only few species from the Varanasi area. Mishra provided short descriptions of the vegetation of Raj Ghat Ravines, Banaras Hindu University, campus and low laying lands and reported 115, 137 and 44 plant species respectively.

The study found that the plants recorded from the site are highly valuable for medicinal uses including diarrhea, dysentery, gonorrhea, leprosy, paralysis, piles, purgative, stomach complaints, ulcer, arthritis, wounds, cholera, diabetes liver complaints, skin diseases, syphilis, throat infections urine complaints, snake bite, body swelling, tumor, malaria, menstrual complaints, rheumatic, skin diseases, swelling, tonic, pulmonary tuberculosis, dog bite, eye diseases, hyperactivity, hydrophobia and lumbago. The study provides sufficient ground to believe that the traditional medicinal practice using native medicinal plants is alive well functioning in the study area. Many communities use wild plant parts for the primary healthcare, due to belief in its effectiveness, lack of modern medicines and medication and poor economic status of people. The treatment of disease with plants and plant products also causes little site effects and is cost effective too.

Keeping the importance of plants in consideration, large numbers of commercially important medicinal plant species are over-exploited by persons involved in the trade. Lack of sustainable harvesting methods, inadequate knowledge about forest management and lack of financial resources are the main causes of over-exploitation, indiscriminate collection and over-exploitation of some commercially important species, and the populations of valuable species are decline.

Man-made extinction of species and habitat degradation are the order of the day. This bio-depletion is due to the exponential geometric growth of human population and man's technological capacity to exploit natural resources in an unsustainable way. Intensive and unrestricted grazing, year after year by multitudes of cattle and goats of local villager, accompanied with spread pilferage from the wild has led to serious decline of medicinal plants in particular and the entire natural environment as whole. More than 95% of the medicinal plant material used by the medicinal plant industry is acquired from the wild more often than not by illegal means.

Conclusion

The area of Varanasi has been settled for millennia, and represents now a large urban environment. Despite dense urbanization, medicinal plants still play a key role in the health care of the local population. Plants commonly used as traditional medicines in rural areas could still be found in the city, and were collected and used by the local population. Local Kavirag and village Vaidyas often collected the medicinal plants from the area of Benares Hindu University campus when they enter for grazing their cattle. The current over-exploitation and soil compaction due to trampling seems to limit the ability of some species to propagate. Therefore, there is immediate need to conserve these important species for sustainable uses for the future. Efforts should be taken to start sustainable cultivation and harvesting programs in the city of Varanasi.

4

Ethnobotany and the Search for Vanishing Knowledge

Before medical researchers paid attention to an old folk tradition and extracted quinine from the bark of cinchona trees, many people died needlessly from malaria. Perhaps similar words will be said about cancer someday . . . unless that cancer cure is never discovered because the tropical tree that produced it became extinct yesterday or the last shaman who knew where to find it died this morning. Does a plant-derived treatment for AIDS or Alzheimer's disease exist today, unknown to modern science, in a previously remote forest slated for bulldozing tomorrow? Whenever I think about it, I smell a vast, ancient library burning. The mid-morning jungle, green on green, full of light and birds, is a peculiar place to think about burning libraries. But a catastrophic loss of knowledge, dwarfing the conflagration at the library of Alexandria, is taking place in the jungles and old-growth forests.

Plant medicines for the body, mind, and soul are becoming extinct at an alarming rate as their host environments are exploited or destroyed. And the people who know how to use the healing plants, the heirs to empirically based, highly pragmatic traditions thousands of years old, are dying too, without leaving successors; those who would have been the apprentices to the remaining elders, the potential heirs of the orally transmitted body of knowledge, are themselves dying or Westernizing even faster than their ancestral habitat is disappearing. An ethnobotanical preserve specializes in plants that are the least studied by Western scientists (and are scantily represented in the botanical gardens), but the most valued by the tribal cultures who use them.

An ethnobotanical preserve isn't easy to build because ethnobotany exists at the uncomfortable convergence of immense destructive forces and cultural taboos: the genocide of indigenous people that is still taking place; the accelerating destruction of the environments that contain the majority of Earth's estimated 250,000 plant species; scientific ignorance of traditional plant-based medicine systems, often based on ethnocentric bias; the abandonment of the search for plant medicines by the U.S. pharmaceutical industry; the taboo against scientific research into plant hallucinogens. The taboo against studying the psychological effects of plant hallucinogens is particularly crippling to those who would preserve and seek to understand traditional knowledge about beneficial plants. First, the people who know the most about traditional botanical medicine, the shamans, claim that their knowledge is derived directly from the plants as well as from their human teachers. And anyone who seeks to understand the dimensions of the shamans' healing system without understanding the place of psychoactive plants is going to miss a vital factor.

Although the usefulness of plants as teachers expands beyond psychedelics to the whole range of medicinal and economic plants, it is counter-productive to ignore the living center of the shamanic plant traditions. Botanical Dimensions was created by Kat and Terence McKenna "to collect, protect, propagate and understand plants of ethnomedical significance and their lore, throughout the world." The heart of the enterprise is a botanical garden on 19 acres of meadow and forest at 2,200 feet on the island of Hawaii, created and nurtured over the past ten years by Terence and Kat, their assistants, volunteers, and network of collectors. The McKennas and a small number of colleagues are striving to save plant species (and something more fragile than plant species) from extinction. The knowledge held by the last of the shamans is a precious resource. In the past, research based on folk traditions led to pharmaceuticals that saved millions of lives.

Gathering such knowledge in the first place must have been a painstaking and hazardous process for early generations of experimental shamans, requiring remarkable bravery as well as ironclad devotion to the experimental method in order to sift through the hundreds of thousands of plants, many of them fatally toxic, to find the ones with specifically useful effects. Which is what generation upon generation of shamans did, from the Himalayas to the Andes. Chavin art from the Peruvian highlands, circa 1300 B.C., depicts the ritual use of the shamanic San Pedro cactus (Trichocereus pachanoi) that is still used as physical and spiritual medicine today.(1) Perhaps a healing tradition over 3,000 years old that is still in use should not be too lightly dismissed. The Ayahuasca cult of Amazonia is of unknown antiquity. Mayan and Aztec art clearly exalt the properties of psilocybin mushrooms. Explicit petroglyphs in North Africa reveal the existence of psychedelic mushroom cults more than 12,000 years ago.

The existence of the dwindling remnants of the living mushroom cult of the Mexican Sierra Mazateca were discovered in the 1950s; prior to Gordon Wasson's discovery of Maria Sabina in Hautla de Jimenez, the antiquity and extent of sacred plant cults was unknown to scientists and scholars of the industrialized world. Western medicine is a few centuries old, and until recently dismissed the mind-body healing aspects of botanical psychedelic shamanism with words like "witch doctor." Nevertheless, there is ample evidence that herbal shamanism was an experimental form of psychosomatic medicine, a form of science as well as a religious subculture. The invisible but precious aspect of these traditions is the body of knowledge acquired by each shaman through a lifetime of learning from plant and human teachers. The pioneering ethnobotanauts who survived their research in do-it-yourself pharmaceutical analysis passed along the best of their knowledge to their apprentices.

A plant-using shaman is far more than a witch doctor who gets wigged out on drugs; he or she is a healer, experimentalist, and psychopomp. The shaman's knowledge was a kind of cultural library for the tribal group. Each shaman learned, applied, and passed along knowledge of botany and bonesetting, hunting lore and agronomy, pharmacy and storytelling, spiritual and social wisdom vital to the welfare of the tribe, knowledge related not only to healing but to warfare, to relocating the village or settling family disputes, to any of the critically important decisions that maintain the life of the culture in relationship to their natural environment. The plant teachers were used for guidance and decision-making and to remain in balance with the natural world. In the past, when Western medical researchers did pay attention to this knowledge, the payoff was spectacular.

As this article is being written, one of the most promising experimental AIDS drugs, known as "GLQ223," is derived from the root of a Chinese plant in the cucumber family. Yet, despite the well-known success of other "folk medicines" such as digitoxin and digoxin (heart failure), ergotamine (migraine), salicin (inflammation and pain), morphine (pain) vincaleukoblastine and leurocristine (Hodgkin's disease and childhood leukemia), and more than 100 other antibiotics, antitumor agents, immune-system stimulants, tranquilizers, sedatives, contraceptives, anaesthetics, laxatives, and pain relievers, the United States has no commercial or government effort to discover and develop new drugs from higher plants. One of the reasons for this dearth of commercial interest in the U.S. is the regulatory structure that makes it preferable for pharmaceutical companies to pursue "rational drug design strategies" in search of new, synthetic (and more easily patentable) drugs; another reason is that drug firms failed in their early attempts at discovering new medicines from plants because of a lack of interdisciplinary cooperation and the lack of inexpensive, portable, accurate bioassay technologies.

All of these obstacles can be surmounted, particularly if the current wave of interest in natural foods and plant medicines raises the economic stakes for the American drug market. And other countries, notably Germany and China, are already engaged in vigorous ethnobotanical R & D. But while the scientific bureaucracies clear up their political differences, and the vendors and regulators stumble toward a policy that might encourage research and preservation, the body of knowledge and the associated biomass are disappearing. Plants have never captured the public imagination the way whales or baby seals do — the plant division of the National Wildlife Federation was created only in recent years, in response to the urgent appeals of ethnobotanist Mark Plotkin.

Trees are the sexiest plants, and while the loss of the great forests continues, it no longer continues unprotested or uncontested. Some organizations are trying to preserve some priceless remainder of the environment in which known useful plants and tens of thousands of undiscovered others still live; other organizations are trying to preserve indigenous peoples and their cultures. But the specific pursuit of ethnobotanical knowledge is a grueling task, and at the heart of it is a subject that happens to be taboo in our culture at this time — direct confrontation with spiritual and medical knowledge through the ingestion of consciousness-expanding plants. As Terence McKenna pointed out, machete in hand, while we walked along the jungle path surrounding the preserve: "No one is preserving this information.

Or precious few of us, anyway. It's professionally dangerous to have anything to do with this information." He was pointing at a brown liana, as thick as my arm in places, coiling its way up tree trunks, limbs, and around itself in heliocentric pilgrimage to the jungle canopy. The "dangerous information" McKenna was mourning encompasses a lot of territory. The vine itself, Banistereopsis caapi, is a key ingredient in the sacramental infusion used by an old medical, religious, psychiatric, and social system — the ayahuasca cult. The little that is known about the psychosocial system that has grown up around the plant over thousands of years is intriguing; legends and anecdotal reports hint at direct perception of knowledge regarding diet, medicine, spiritual growth and personal conduct — the plant itself as the teacher/healer/psychopomp. Other persistent rumors concern "shared states of mind" and self-diagnostic capabilities. In the ayahuasca cults, the medicine, the plant, and the teacher are all the same entity. McKenna also was referring to the incalculably larger collective loss of knowledge regarding thousands of medicinal, economic, and spiritual plants that is taking place. The knowledge that is slipping away from us concerns the foundations of human well-being — health, sanity, imagination, social harmony. And plant-based medicine is not simply a New Age nostrum (although the best place for an American to obtain herbal remedies is the nearest upscale natural-foods boutique). According to the World Health Organization, approximately 70 percent of the world's population rely on the use of plant extracts within the context of "traditional medicine" as their primary source of health care. At the same time, American consumers paid more than $8 billion in 1985 for prescriptions whose active constituents were extracted from plants.

In the early 1970s, with no concerted effort by any pharmaceutical company, government, or international body, Terence McKenna was recruited directly by the plants themselves to export, preserve, and propagate them. A University of California graduate with an interdisciplinary degree in conservation of natural resources, he set out in the first of several South American expeditions in search of rare ethnobotanical specimens. An expedition to a remote tributary of the Putomayo river in the Colombian Amazon led to his first experiences with the mushroom Stropharia cubensis, which he and his brother Dennis succeeded in cultivating after several years of effort. In 1976 he married another enthusiastic amateur ethnobotanist, Kathleen Harrison, and by 1977 they had found the land in Hawaii — three hours by machete from the nearest road — and started moving their specimens there. Kat was in Thailand at the time I visited, in search of the fabled kratom.

Terence and his charming young son Finn took me for morning walks along the trail that encircled their property, pointing out specimens of the more than 60 imported species that were growing there at the time. Shortly after I returned to the mainland, 50 new species arrived from South America, and through an arrangement Kat had made with a botanical garden in Bangkok, new Asian specimens began to arrive. The transplantation process is laborious, because the soil layer is very thin. For each specimen, a hole has to be dug in the rocky lava soil, and soil amendments have to be hauled in and mixed, before the plant can be placed in the ground. Terence explained the process of obtaining a plant, while we walked through the heart of Botanical Dimensions. "When you bring out plants, you bring out dozens of plants at a time, consisting of many species and many specimens of each species," he began. "You need a phytosanitary certificate, which you obtain from the U.S. Department of Agriculture. But you need a different collection of papers before you get to that point. The process begins when you read about a plant of interest in some ethnobotanical paper, or hear a rumor of a plant. Before you mount an expedition, you need letters of support from a botanist at one or more universities, attesting to your status as a skilled, if amateur, ethnobotanist.

If you know what you are doing, this should be possible to do; keep in mind that ethnobotany is one science where many of the major contributions have been made by well-informed amateurs." As McKenna explained it, the advance paperwork is just the first step in a bureaucratic labyrinth: "After obtaining seeds, cuttings, or (preferably), root stock of the sought-after plants, we arrive in the capital city of Country X, preparing to return home.

After insuring that proper botanical identification is provided to smooth the export and import process, our first call is on the botany department of the national university, where we give half of our specimens to the chairman of the department. He, in turn, writes us a friendly cover letter which we take over to their plant export people, who then, after delays, agree that we can depart with all this stuff. And then they stamp it, issue reams of paper about it, and we fly out. We then arrive at Los Angeles or Miami with this carton of living plants; we leave the ordinary customs processes and go directly to the Department of Agriculture people, who gas all the plants, wash away any soil that may be clinging to their roots, and give them back to us, somewhat the worse for wear.

Then we rewrap them, repackage them, and air express them to their destination, where they are immediately fed vitamins, put into potting soil, and babied along. Perhaps half the original specimens survive this process, which can take up to a year. Then we get to find out if they can actually adapt to the new environment, a process that can take several years, and if they thrive we propagate them." Although a network of botanists, anthropologists, chemists, psychotherapists, and psychologists are trying (discreetly) to learn something about the use of these plants and the nature of their active ingredients, the taboos against overt psychedelic research make it difficult to organize the kind of broad interdisciplinary effort needed to approach this body of knowledge and medicinal substances. Botanical Dimensions reminds me of the monasteries of the Dark Ages in Europe, in which monks carefully copied manuscripts they didn't understand, century after century, keeping the information together until the Renaissance lifted the taboos on classical wisdom. "We're just trying to keep the plants alive through the current dark age, until a future society, more enlightened than the present one, takes an unbiased look at their potential," Terence said, back at the shadehouse, after our first walk through the property. The great green library is burning. But at least some determined amateurs are trying to save a remnant of the old knowledge before it all goes up in smoke or smothers in concrete.

5

Ethics in Herbal Medicine

INTRODUCTION

Herbal system of medicine has been practiced since historical times and traces its roots to ancient civilizations. Although, we define alternative systems of healing as subjects that are not taught in medical schools, it is worthwhile to mention that before the availability of synthetic drugs, plant-based remedies formed the basis of primary healthcare system. Herbal infusion, decoction and tinctures were house-hold remedies for common ailments. In the Indian context, the house hold remedies are better known as *dadi ma ke nuskhe* (elderly formulations).

Traditional medicine includes certain health approaches and practices incorporating the use of herbs, metals or diet restrictions or life style changes, with a view to diagnose, prevent or treat diseases. Recently, the World Health Organization (W.H.O.) introduced CAM (Complementary and Alternative) health practices in various parts of the world. Broadly speaking, all systems defined under CAM come under Traditional Medicine. In other words, complementary and alternative systems are an off shoot of traditional medicine. Alternative medicine includes replacement of one system with another. Complementary health practices include adding one system of medicine as adjunct to another.

Ayurveda, Siddha, Yunani, Homeopathy, Naturopathy, Reflexology, Aromatherapy, Alexander's technique, Western Medical

Herbalism and Traditional Chinese Medicine (T.C.M.) represent some popular traditional systems of medicine. All these systems have been practiced in the past with considerable success. T.C.M. has made tremendous advances in terms of modern scientific research, and according to latest studies it contributes 80 % of the annual turnover of the total herbal drug industry.

Ayurveda, Siddha, Yunani, Homeopathy, Aromatherapy, Western Medical Herbalism and Traditional Chinese Medicine are largely dependent on medicinal plants for preparing formulations. In our view, herbal medicine is a broad term covering all traditional, alternative and complementary systems of medicine utilizing plants.

RENAISSANCE OF HERBAL MEDICINE

Herbal medicine is making a dramatic comeback. Studies done across the world have demonstrated increasing awareness about herbal medicine among the general population. According to World Health Organisation, majority of the people living in rural belt are dependent on medicinal plants for curing common diseases. Further, the importance of herbal medicine can be assessed by the fact that 60% of synthetic drugs have roots in medicinal plants.

Several factors are responsible for the comeback of herbal medicine. Drug resistance seems to be the prime cause. Cost-effectiveness is another factor where herbal drugs score over synthetic drugs. The efficacy of some herbal products is beyond doubt, the most recent examples being *Artemisia annua* (i.e., artemesinin: wormwood derivative used to target cancers), *Silybum marianum* (i.e., silymarin: seeds of the milk thistle effective in treating diseases of the liver) and *Taxus brevifolia* (i.e., taxols: pacific yew derivative that exhibits antimitotic activity and is used for treating refractory tumors).

At the same time, it must be argued that old sayings like 'herbal drugs are safe and can be consumed over a period of time without side-effects boast of any scientific proof. Herbal-synthetic drug interactions are major challenge for practitioners. Hepatotoxicity and nephrotoxicity associated with certain medicinal herbs pose major health problem. Post-operative bleeding associated with herbal remedies is another cause of concern.

It can be said that there is rise as well as fall in popularity of herbal medicines in recent times. Extracts/drugs prepared from medicinal plants having definite mechanism of action are respected among allopathic physicians. Herbal drugs are of much value in chronic and degenerative ailments of the body. There are many reports that some patients, after utilizing herbal formulations over a period of time feel that they are therapeutically useless. In our view, there is an obvious difference between rigorously researched product and cheaply/unethically promoted product.

HERBAL CLINICAL PRACTICE

The herbal system of medicine is alternatively known as medical herbalism or botanical medicine. Recently phytotherapy has been used as a popular alternative for plant-based formulations

In older days, knowledge of herbalism was based on experience. Hardly any work was done on documentation of plant-based remedies. Practical classes were the major weapon of acquiring knowledge on herbalism. With a passage of time, the need of documentation was felt and several texts were written. Majority of traditional systems of medicine have their own texts. These texts, once upon a time, were popularly known as Materia Medica, a term that has largely been replaced by pharmacognosy.

Herbal clinical practice is largely based on experience of an herbalist or natural medicine physician. Herbalists tend to prepare their own medicines, therefore, in the majority of cases, the patient does not know about the nature of the drug. In Ayurvedic practice, a majority of the Ayurvedachrayas dispense there own formulations. Now the trend is changing. With major pharmaceutical companies diversifying in phyto-pharmaceuticals manufacturing, practitioners have developed interest in writing prescriptions.

Following factors may be held responsible for limitations of herbal clinical practice:

Non-availability of medicines: Herbal prescriptions range from single herb to poly-herbal formulations. In case of writing herbal prescriptions, availability of medicines is necessary. Non-availability of medicines at drug stores is another limitation of herbal/Ayurvedic practice.

Expiry date on labels: Lack of information of expiry date on the bottle is ruining herbal clinical practice. This also impacts the therapeutic efficacy of the medicine. Owing to non-availability of medicines and lack of expiry date, the CAM practitioners believe in dispensing medicines on there own.

Variety of medicinal plants/drugs: Another factor that limits the scope of herbal/CAM practice is the number of medicinal plants mentioned in respective pharmacopeias. In Ayurveda, 850 medicinal plants are actively used for creating formulations.

Vague health claims: Most of the practitioners of Ayurveda opt for allopathic practice after graduate studies. Doctors with postgraduate studies, opt for teaching professions or industry. Limited number of Ayurvedic physicians settles in urban territory. It is a sorry state of affairs that most of the people who have opened Ayurvedic/herbal clinics are professionally untrained. The situation gets complicated when 'self-styled' physicians make claims for permanently curing intractable diseases like AIDS, hepatitis and cancer. This is violation of the Magical Remedy Act.

Adulterated/spurious medications: Several reports have been published regarding mixing of synthetic drugs like corticosteroids and pain-killers in herbal prescriptions. This has harmed the belief of many people in the alternative system of medicine.

Medicinal plant identification in Ayurveda: In Ayurveda, several medicinal plants have controversial identities, and it is important to establish their proper botanical identity.

Example 1: Let us cite the example of Ashtavarga, an important ingredient of composite Ayurvedic formulation. Ashtavarga is an important ingredient of various classical Ayurvedic formulations like Chavyanprasha. Ashtavarga has been assigned various medicinal properties by ancient Materia Medica dealing with Ayurveda. The eight plants mentioned under Ashtavarga are considered to be medicinal plants of controversial origin, despite the fact that work has been done on their botanical identity.

Table 1. Eight medicinal plants used in Ashtavarga, composite Ayurvedic formulation.

S.No.	Ayurvedic name	Botanical name	Family	Part used
1.	Jivaka	*Malaxis muscifera* (Lindl.) Kuntze	Orchidaceae	Bulb
2.	Rishbhaka	*Malaxis acuminta* D.Don	Orchidaceae	Pseudo-bulb
3.	Meda	*Polygonatum verticillatum* (L.) All.	Polygonaceae	Rhizome
4.	Mahameda	*Polygonatum cirrhifolium* (Wall.) Royle	Polygonaceae	Rhizome
5.	Kakoli	*Roscoea procera* Wall.	Zingiberaceae	Root
6.	Kshira-Kakoli	1. *Fritillaria royeli* Hook.f 2. *Lilium polphyllum* D.Don	Liliaceae	Root
7.	Riddhi	*Habenaria intermedia* D.Don	Orchidaceae	Root
8.	Vriddhi	*Habenaria edgeworthii* Hook.f. ex Collett.	Orchidaceae	Root

Most of the Ayurvedic drugs manufacturing companies using Ashtavarga in formulations are depicting botanical name mentioned in the table. However, literature search reveals that certain medical plants of family Ascelpiadaceae are possible representatives of Kakoli, Kshira-kakoli and Meda.

Table 2. Alternative representatives of certain ingredients of Ashtavarga.

S.No.	Ayurvedic name	Botanical name	Family
1.	Kakoli	*Gymnema balsamicum*	Ascelpiadaceae
2.	Kshira-kakoli	*Gymnema lactiferum* (L.) R.Br. ex Schult.	Ascelpiadaceae
3.	Meda	*Gymnema aurantiaca*	Ascelpiadaceae

As already discussed, Chavyanprasha is a hot-selling product in the Indian market. It is considered to be panacea for treatment of chronic respiratory ailments, thanks to its tonic effect. Since Ashtavarga is a significant ingredient of Chavyanprasha, it is essential that exact plants be identified in the manufacture of the composite formulation.

Example 2: Pashanbheda is another example worth mentioning. It is a well-known lithontriptic (stone-dissolving) drug of Ayurveda. The following plants are used as pasanbheda in different parts of India:

Table 3. Medicinal plants used for ancient drug Pasahanbheda.

S.no	Botanical name	Family
1.	*Aerva lanata* Juss.ex Schult.	Amaranthaceae
2.	*Bergenia ligulata* (Wall.) Engl.	Saxifragaceae
3.	*Bridelia crenulata* Roxb.	Euphorbiaceae
4.	*Bryophyllum calycinum* Salisb.	Crassulaceae
5.	*Coleus amboinicus* Lour.	Lamiaceae
6.	*Decalepis arayalpathra* Joseph & Chandrasekharan	*Periplocaceae*
7.	*Homonoia riporia* Lour.	Euphorbiaceae
8.	*Rotula aquatica* Lour.	Boraginaceae

Lack of awareness among physicians: Recently, several clinical trials with Ayurvedic/herbal drugs have been published in reputed journals. As an instance, guggul is widely used in Ayurveda in the treatment of obesity. Animal and human trials have suggested that guggul is useful for reducing high blood-cholesterol and triglycerides. This is perfect example of bridging the gap between traditional and modern medicine. A book like PDR should be part of all natural medicine clinics.

Lack of awareness among patients: We need to educate the patients seeking alternative medicine advice. We need to tell them categorically about the nature of herbal drugs. Herbal remedies are not magical bullets and have nothing to do with emergency conditions. However, chronic and degenerative diseases do respond to herbal remedies. While buying Ayurvedic products, the patients should always look for the label indicating 'metals with permissible limits'. They should also ensure the originality of the medication.

Self-medication: Self medication with herbal remedies is increasing becoming popular. Most of the herbal remedies like Garlic, St. John's wort, Ginkgo and Spirulina are commonly available over the counter remedies in US and UK. In India, medicinal plants used in Ayurveda are available in capsule or tablet form. This free sale should be controlled as there are increased reports of herbal-synthetic drug interactions in recent times. The patient should always try to consult a qualified physician before consuming any medication.

Bias against herbal medicine: False propaganda against herbal medicine should be discontinued immediately. We do not wish to rebuke or promote any system of medicine. Herbal system of medicine should be accepted with an open mind and its advantages and disadvantages should be kept in mind.

OTHER SIDE OF HERBAL MEDICINE

Herbal medicine has several advantages:

Source of lead compounds: Medicinal plants are significant source of drugs and new chemical entities (NCEs). Phytochemistry (chemical composition) and phyto-pharmacology are rapidly making progress as far as research and development is concerned. In our view, medicinal phytochemistry should be a distinct subject in syllabus of herbal medicine. Several phytochemicals have been isolated from medicinal plants and screened for applied research. Several companies maintain natural products libraries. Drugs derived from herbal source can play a significant role in future healthcare system, keeping in mind emergence of drug resistance.

Cost-effectiveness: Herbal drugs are cheaper, if readily available. Many drugs have been synthesised from intermediates obtained from plant source. Bromhexine was derived from alkaloid vasicine isolated from *Adathoda vasica* Nees. The drug is popular anti-tussive (cough-suppressant).

Side-effect profile: Herbal remedies, if purified according to methods mentioned in pharmacopeias and prepared according to the drug formulary, are relatively non-toxic. It is generally understood herbal remedies are benign and free from side-effects. However, evidence suggests that herbal remedies may pose side –effects, if consumed without professional advice. With onset of scientific research in herbal medicine, data for side-effects of herbal is accumulating. Based on herbal clinical practice, it can be said that side effect profile of herbals is however less as compared to synthetic drugs.

CONCLUSION

With increasing number of patients consulting herbal medicine practitioners, herbal clinical practice will be of more relevance in future. The need of the hour is to take herbal medicine with an open mind. Herbal product claims, supported by scientific evidence should be used in clinical practice with confidence. This will enhance the physician-patient compliance and provide the much needed support to herbal clinical practice.

6

Bioprospecting the African Renaissance: The New Value of Muthi

This chapter gives an overview of anthropological research on bioprospecting in general and of available literature related to bioprospecting particularly in South Africa. It points out how new insights on value regimes concerning plant-based medicines may be gained through further research and is meant to contribute to a critical discussion about the ethics of Access and Benefit Sharing (ABS). In South Africa, traditional healers, plant gatherers, petty traders, researchers and private investors are assembled around the issues of standardization and commercialization of knowledge about plants. This coincides with a nation-building project which promotes the revitalization of local knowledge within the so called African Renaissance.

A social science analysis of the transformation of so called Traditional Medicine (TM) may shed light onto this renaissance by tracing social arenas in which different regimes of value are brought into conflict. When medicinal plants turn into assets in a national and global economy, they seem to be manipulated and transformed in relation to their capacity to promote health, their market value, and their potential to construct new ethics of development. In this context, the translation of socially and culturally situated local knowledge about *muthi* into global pharmaceuticals creates new forms of agency as well as new power differentials between the different actors involved.

BIOVALUE IN THE AFRICAN RENAISSANCE

A growing demand for herbal medicines in North America and Europe as well as epidemics like Malaria, Tuberculosis and HIV/AIDS in Sub-Sahara African have created an expanding market for indigenous herbal medicines. Traditional healers, plant gatherers, petty traders, research institutions and private corporations have assembled around the issues of standardization and commercialization of local knowledge about plants. In South Africa this coincides with a nation-building project, which promotes the revitalization of local knowledge in the so called "African Renaissance". The idea of such renaissance is as old as the Pan-Africanist movement and its struggle for a regeneration of the continent after slavery and colonialism. More recently, it was proclaimed by Thabo Mbeki's presidential campaigns as synonymous to a "second liberation struggle" for self-discovery, democratization and economic development. There is reason to assume that the transformation of so called Traditional Medicine (TM) sheds light onto this renaissance by indicating how different regimes of value are brought into conflict. Indeed, the translation of socially and culturally situated local knowledge into global pharmaceuticals creates new forms of agency as well as new power differentials between corporate investors, scientists, plant gatherers, and traditional healers. The present article alludes to the transformation of TM in South Africa by giving an overview of key moments in bioprospecting, the "exploration of biodiversity for commercially valuable genetic and biochemical resources". It will thereby trace social arenas in which plant based medicines have been assigned biovalue.

Catherine Waldby first introduced the concept of biovalue to designate the relationship between the promotion of health, the production of capital and the question of ethics in the context of human tissue and stem cell research.

It is generated through the manipulation of biological processes in the laboratory and yields therapeutic as well as monetary revenue. Furthermore, as emphasized by Novas and Rose it is simultaneously commercial and ethical. In the present review, the notion of biovalue will depict the assignment of value to genetic material derived from indigenous medical plants. Although plants markedly differ from human stem cells similar dynamics seem to be at stake. Following Waldby, we are able to discern at least three main points of relevance to bioprospecting in the African Renaissance, emerging from a review of existing policy papers, legal frameworks, and academic research. When medicinal plants turn into assets in a national and global economy they become manipulated and transformed in relation to their capacity to promote health, their market value, and their potential to construct a new ethics of development. Before addressing these three aspects, I will first of all point to some anthropological work relevant for future studies on bioprospecting in society. I then give an overview of literature on bioprospecting within Social and Cultural Anthropology. Finally, the paper will be point out how new insights on value regimes on plant-based medicines may be gained through further research.

MEDICAL PLURALISMS, TECHNOLOGY AND SCIENCE

The process of enlightenment, globalization, modernity or post-modernity has been characterized by accelerating social change in the face of ambiguity, fragmentation and a quest for new certainties. Human experience becomes tangled by anonymous flows of capital, technologies, goods, people, images and ideas that may restrain at the same time as they may expand subjects' agency. While there is a growing number of studies about the effects of this process at large, few concentrate on the transformation of plant-based traditional medicines and even less do so in Africa. Teleological assumptions made by Modernization Theory have been challenged by research in Medical Anthropology. Accordingly, information and education based on "scientific facts" do not automatically result in a replacement of so called "traditional beliefs". While some local medical treatments vanish over time others may be transformed, revitalized or reinvented. Furthermore, it has been documented how subjects choose therapies and etiology eclectically, thereby generating new systems of signification. In this sense, the impact of biomedical science and technology results in medical pluralisms and the hybridization of medical practice.

If this is the case with contemporary African medical systems, it is vital to analyze how the appropriation of new practices takes place among the different actors involved and what new significations and meanings are produced by medical pluralism. However, biomedicine is not just another link in a harmonic alignment of health care providers. Dominant discourses based on cosmopolitan notions of health introduced by international development agencies, multinational corporations and state institutions may well conflict with the ones adopted by rural plant collectors, petty traders or traditional healers. It has been argued that in order to reach beyond a mere documentation of medical pluralisms, the process of signification must be deciphered by a thorough analysis of power relations. These become particularly salient in the field of property rights. The Anthropology of Law has long addressed cultural variation in property regimes, trends towards flexible dispute resolution instead of rights based decision-making and the local appropriation of legal forms in multiple settings.

These studies have hardly been linked to research on bioprospecting in society and on the role of the biosciences in the negotiation of property rights in developing countries. It has in fact long been argued that science in general assumes a hegemonic position through the construction of its object. Theorizing in the anthropology and sociology of knowledge emphasizes that the externalized products of human activity attain the character of objectivity through a dialectical relationship between humans and the social world. Ethnography has shown that there is no straightforward trajectory from laboratory research and the discovery of so called facts to medical technologies and their rational implementation in the social field. Beyond the physical level of biomedical disease, the process of signification is tied to the specific interests of the actors involved. Calling for a suspension of a conceptual nature/culture divide ethnographic studies of laboratory practice contend that artifacts themselves are involved in the construction of heterogeneous actor-networks of humans and non-human "actants".

On the other hand, anthropological analysis of medicine, science and technology also went beyond epistemological issues and analyzed modes of commodification of life and the emergence of new forms of biopolitical government in the field of genetic resources derived from animals and humans. Frequently, the artifacts of research and development are legitimated and disseminated along powerful global allegiances and social networks rather than being product of neutral reasoning based on natural cause and effect. In this context, the ethnographic study of pharmaceuticals and their biographies has become a promising new field of inquiry that, however, has hardly targeted herbal medicines. Future research will have to include more inquiries into the enclosure of knowledge for the purpose of drug development concerned with genetic or biochemical resources derived from indigenous medical plants. Some relevant examples of anthropological research done in this field are particularly concerned with bioprospecting.

BIOPROSPECTING AND "BIOPIRACY" IN INTERNATIONAL PERSPECTIVE

To date ethnographic studies concerning the process of bioprospecting have primarily focused on the Americas where major bioprospecting agreements were established between the U.S.-based International Cooperative Biodiversity Group (ICBG) and Latin American universities from the early 1990s onwards. In this context, some anthropologists started to suggest that the inclusion of local knowledge into national and international patent law is incompatible with local cosmologies and may ultimately inflict "symbolic violence" upon indigenous cultures. Others have emphasized that these communities are not only passive victims of globalization but rather selectively appropriate cosmopolitan discourses about intellectual property rights for the pursuit of their own interest. It has also been pointed out that the struggle for indigenous rights can even have racist undertones that for the sake of ethno-national endeavors, depict culture as static and unchanging. Such essentialist understandings often result in claims to the "copyright of culture". For Brown, the enclosure of knowledge however, bears the risk of putting an end to science, human progress and even democracy. In another worst-case scenario, bioprospecting could contribute to conflict between different ethnic groups or even nation states that claim ownership to a genetic resource as well as to internal social disintegration of communities.

The latter seems to be true especially when certain factions are externally appointed to be representative of an imagined community although they do not reflect the opinion of the majority of people concerned. The role of NGOs in this process may vary from generating exaggerated expectations about potential benefits through commercialization of IK to an emphasis on its devastating effects. So-called non-profit organizations may even foreclose rights recognition by mediating the interest of multinational corporations. NGOs can nevertheless bring entire bioprospecting programs to halt through accusations of biopiracy or theft of IK. This may be the case even though local resource providers haven't given their mandate to do so. With regard to this problem, it has been claimed that the governance of potentially collaborating indigenous societies is the key to successful benefit-sharing and must therefore be strengthened through capable authorizing institutions as well as a "culture of responsible research".

Critics within anthropology have questioned the notion of biopiracy as non-contractual collection and use of resources as a useful analytical category for it is itself based on an understanding of authorship that underlies the very expropriation of indigenous resources by powerful global actors. From this perspective, benefit-sharing agreements contribute to the construction of bounded communities. Through appropriation from the public domain intellectual property is extended by "closing" agricultural commons whose origin in reality is ambiguous. Cori Hayden's analysis of a bilateral benefit-sharing agreement between the U.S. and Mexico suggests that bio-artifacts contain, reproduce, and represent people's interests, thereby shaping social relationships for each plant collected. In this sense, bioprospecting makes "nature go public" since it generates new audiences for scientific "facts" among private investors and local communities alike. The designation of benefit-recipients whether scientists or local interlocutors whom they are to recruit, creates incentives "to value their resources in ways imagined by project founders and architects". At stake are new forms of governance that produce human subjectivities and natural objects which conceptualize themselves or become conceptualized by idioms of the neoliberal market.

Medicinal plants are not only passive objects of scientific reason; from the perspective of Actor-Network-Theory mentioned above, they attract and connect different human and non-human actors. Through bioprospecting in society the emergent networks are not only constructed in relation to scientific knowledge production, but also in relation to prospective plant producers, private investors, and holders of local knowledge about plants. In this context we can concur with Franklin in arguing that bioprospecting draws nature and its so-called stakeholders into globally emergent forms of biocapital. As pointed out by Sunder Rajan biocapital is a system of exchanges in the life-sciences that leads to an "implosion" of epistemology and political economy. It generates a "hype" around potential medicines that attracts venture capital and creates a speculative marketplace. As such, it is not necessarily based on the actual needs of patients but on the anticipation of future consumers who eventually, may generate high profits. Before turning to the global marketplace created through bioprospecting, I will first of all address its relevance for the promotion of health in South Africa more broadly.

BIOPROSPECTING AND THE PROMOTION OF HEALTH

The transformation of indigenous medical plants has been recently seen as prerequisite for effective health promotion including the reduction of poverty. Whereas under colonialism, health and African tradition were seen as rather contradictory, today there is a revived interest in the way in which so-called Indigenous Knowledge Systems (IKS) can be made applicable for public health. The World Bank's Indigenous Knowledge Program defines IKS as "problem solving strategies for local communities" to achieve the Millennium Development Goals, to promote the sustainable management of resources, to enhance health care and to fight HIV/AIDS.

The World Health Organization has a particular interest in Traditional Medicine, the evaluation of its safety and efficacy and its integration into national healthcare systems. The emphasis on local knowledge among international development organizations partly stems from past experience in ineffective top-down driven technical interventions and a general move toward a discourse on "empowerment" and "participation". The latter have been promoted in view of reducing costs for health care in resource poor settings by transferring more responsibility to the target population itself. The extent to which the search for commercially valuable genetic resources in Southern Africa is tied to new modes of biopolitical government through public health has not yet been addressed through social science research. Indeed, the search for indigenous herbal medicines in South Africa seems to be part of a larger nation-building project called African Renaissance which implicitly draws upon local knowledge, the life-sciences, and the counties' rich biodiversity.

Lund argues that the architects of the new South Africa draw on a long-standing tradition of using biological analogies to interpret social phenomena and to promote national causes. After Apartheid the government took recourse to rhetoric around "healing the nation" using metaphors previously used in colonial and apartheid discourse. Currently, the promotion of South Africa's vitality through bioprospecting takes place within a larger project of self-discovery and the revitalization of African culture coupled with an investment into the life-sciences. President Mbeki, in his well-known African Renaissance statement, emphasizes that "the colonizers sought to enslave the African mind and to destroy the African soul", therefore "the beginning of our rebirth as a continent must be our own rediscovery of our soul".

Since then, much effort has been put into stimulating the contribution of IKS to health and development. The South African IKS policy aims at promoting a positive African identity by the affirmation of African cultural values and the development of services provided by holders of IK, especially in the field of Traditional Medicine. It further maintains that the role of indigenous knowledge in the creation of economic wealth must be strengthened and indigenous knowledge should be "used together with modern biotechnology in the pharmaceutical and other sectors to increase the rate of innovation". Considering South Africa's rich biodiversity, the connection between a "healthy nation" and biology is metaphoric as it is material. Roughly, 700 plant species are used and traded for medical purpose outside the formal biomedical system. The local knowledge, including notions of health and healing, attached to them is currently being transformed.

In South Africa publicly funded research institutions have a marked interest in the commercialization of plant-based medicines purified of cultural and social derivates. All major South African universities have botany or biochemistry departments that engage in bioprospecting activities concerning TM; the same is true for large research institutions like the Medical Research Council (MRC) or the Council for Scientific and Industrial Research (CSIR). It is hoped that prospecting and the commercial cultivation of medical plants will yield new employment opportunities at the rural level and cost-effective drugs against regionally prevalent diseases.

In this context, the promotion of health seems to be tied to the enclosure of knowledge about plants. This enclosure however equates local knowledge with information relevant for bioprospecting. The National Patents Act was amended to include a definition of traditional knowledge as "knowledge that an indigenous community has regarding the use of a biological or genetic resource". Indeed, the cosmopolitan language of the life-sciences favors certain aspects being immediately compatible with analyzing plant based medicines in the laboratory, while neglecting others that may still be meaningful to local producers, distributors, patients and healers. In South Africa approximately 350.000 Traditional Healers offer medicinal plants to 60–80% of the population. Wreford argues that while healers are quite interested in partnerships and associations with biomedicine, the enthusiasm is hardly reciprocated. They are expected to adapt to biomedicine in a "unidirectional project".

Indeed, mutual understanding between traditional healers, state officials, and scientists seems to be rather limited. Once highlighted by Ngubane, the distinction between herbalist or *inyanga* and diviner or *sangoma* is now widely endorsed by the state. For research institutions *inyangas* are the main representatives of local knowledge due to their assumed compatibility with Western epistemology. Although patients hardly distinguish them from *sangomas*, the latter have been confined to the realm of religion and belief. Such categorization seems to deceptive considering the complex interrelationships between the physical, the social and the spiritual world, established through African healers' diagnosis and treatment. This becomes salient in the concept of *muthi*, which derives from the Nguni root *-thi* and signifies tree. It refers to a substance or mixture of different substances primarily derived from plant material and processed in a way either to achieve positive effects of healing, cleansing and protection from evil forces or negative ones of witchcraft, misfortune and ill-health. A study of Xhosa chemists in Eastern Cape Province by Cocks and Moller found that almost one third of medicines were purchased for "personal well being" and "cultural purpose", like warding off evil spirits and to bring good luck.

However, clear-cut distinctions between those remedies that fall in the realm of culture and those falling into that of life-science must be treated with caution. There are epistemological similarities and differences between indigenous and biomedical notions of herbal medicine. Ashforth explains this issue vividly by illustrating how from the emic point of view, *muthi* may be activated by spirits, may be applied from spatial distance and does not necessarily have to enter the body. From this perspective, *muthi* is inherently ambiguous since it can be understood either as medicine or poison according to the moral interpretation of intentions involved in its application. Without constructing a simple binary opposition between "local tradition" and "global science" it is safe to say that some interfaces and conflicts are likely to result from divergent ideas about *muthi* and its health promoting properties which are being prospected.

The Generation of Monetary Value

With the advent of market-exchange medicinal plants, the knowledge attached to them is not only valued for healing but also for commercial purpose. African medicinal plants have entered the speculative marketplace of biocapital. The importance of investment in the "high growth" sectors of biotechnology and phytomedicine have been addressed in the founding document of the New Partnership for Africa's Development (NEPAD) and later been specified by the African Biosciences Initiative.

Particularly in South Africa, there is a substantial market for plant based medicines. Ten years ago plant species traded for medical use already made up 20.000 tons of plant material with an estimated annual value of 38 Mil. US$. The *muthi* trade is mostly based on a "hidden economy" of self-dependent plant gatherers, street vendors and healers, which forms part of income generating strategies of rural households and especially low income women. Considered as an untapped source for economic development, the *muthi* market is difficult to approach by state institutions and pharmaceutical companies. For successful commercialization of plant based medicine on a national and global scale, property rights are deemed prerequisite. The World Trade Organization's (WTO) Agreement on Trade Related Aspects of Intellectual Property Rights (TRIPS) protects inventions of legal persons based on novelty, non-obviousness and innovation. The agreement states that member parties may exclude plants and essential biological processes from patentability but obliges them to provide for the protection of plant varieties either by patents or by the maintenance of ex-situ plant collections or a combination thereof (Art. 27/3).

One of the first efforts to establish a national collection of biomedically valuable plants in South Africa dates back to the 1990s when a company called Noristan Laboratories donated a database to the University of Cape Town's Pharmacology Department. The Traditional Medicines Project (TRAMED) was subsequently criticized by an US based group called "People's Health Alliance Rejecting Medical Authoritarianism Prejudice and Conspiratorial Tyranny" (PHARMAPACT) for illegitimately disclosing local knowledge. New information and communication technologies enabled the NGO to spread the concern of a TM sell-out. Militant accusations and some media coverage around "biopiracy" culminated in the late 1990s when the South African Medicines and Medical Devices Regulatory Authority Act was authorized (MDRA 1998).

For the first time all medicines, including TM had to be registered with the Medicines Control Council and could only be sold with disclosure of their ingredients. While some argued that the regulation of TM would be vital for the safety and efficacy of treatments, others maintained that TM could not be evaluated in biomedical terms. Furthermore, it was feared the new legislation served the more subtle purpose of controlling economic revenues gained from plant medicines. Sipho Mndaweni, former president of the Interim Coordinating Committee of Traditional Practitioners in South Africa (ICCTP), was one of the first to complain that "traditional healers and vendors may end up being squeezed out of the market", insisting that "we won't see a cent of the vast profits they will make, even though people will buy these goods thinking it's the same as what we do". Although submissions were directed to Parliament to claim control over the trademark Traditional Medicine, the trend since is largely driven by attempts to standardize TM in biomedical terms. Internet-platforms like TRAMED have to some extent substituted *sangomas* and *inyangas* as primary source of knowledge about endemic medical plants as candidates for bioprospecting.

In fact, several Southern African plant varieties that have been previously patented in North America and Europe are now being protected under TRIPS. An exemplary case is the patenting of a purified extract from *Harpagophytum procumbens*, assigned by the German company Finkelberg, a leading producer of plant extracts for the pharmaceutical industry. The substance may be used for the preparation of medications for the treatment of asthma, inflammatory conditions of the gastro intestinal tract or diseases of the rheumatic type. The healing properties of the plant that came to be known as devil's claw have been recognized by the Khoisan people of the Kalahari long before they were primarily divulged to a German colonial soldier in the late 19th century. However, the originators of the medicine were neither addressed through patent negotiations nor did they benefit from the large commercial success of the drug in Germany where it turned into the third most frequently used natural drug of all. Currently, corporations like Ratiopharm or Hexal offer a 50 g extract of devil's claw in tablet form for roughly 25 Euros. According to the German Church Development Service San plant gatherers in Namibia are at best paid 30–40 cents per kilogram of dried tubers, while others are hired for no other payment than food and drink.

A more recent case of controversy concerns the patenting of extracts from *Pelargonium sidoides* and *Pelargonium reniforme* by the company ISO Arzneimittel. The former is predominantly found in the South Africa's Eastern Cape while the latter is endemic throughout the cape regions and KwaZuluNatal as well as to Lesotho. There is growing bioscientific evidence of the antibacterial, antifungal and antitubercular activity of plant extracts. Although *Pelargomium* has been used as medicinal plant for a variety of infectious disease by Xhosa, Zulu and Basotho people for many generations, this was neither acknowledged by the new patent holders nor by South African companies which market the drug already for more than a decade without claims to intellectual property. Officials from ISO Arzneimittel still hold that they won't challenge their South African competitors. However, according to the African Centre for Biosafety, no ABS agreement has been established in the forefront of the two patents, granted in 2003 and 2005, respectively. So far, local resource providers have seen little benefit of bioprospecting, not only in the case of *Pelargonium* which is commonly used to treat HIV related infections in the region.

An assessment of the overall use of biological resources in South Africa conducted by the South African Biodiversity Institute (SANBI) found that permits were mostly applied for the collection of biological resources for "research purpose". However, frequently collectors did not participate in the "drawing up" of Material Transfer Agreements or Memoranda of Understanding. About 50% of the resource suppliers reported that there was no mechanism to share benefits; the other 50% claimed to have received some incentives like immediate cash or copies of reports. The above mentioned examples may indicate a failed African Renaissance since the "re-discovery" of the medicines seems to have neither added value to economic development nor led to enhancement of health care in the region. To date, there is little data available on the impact of bioprospecting on "hidden economies" in South Africa. In how far the generation of surplus and the assignment of monetary value to plant-based medicines is something new for plant gatherers and healers as well as for bioscientist still remains to be seen. The impact of biocapital on moral economies of reciprocal gift exchange and/or redistribution which might still be prevalent in rural regions has not been paid much attention either.

The Generation of Ethical Value

We have to take cognisance of the fact that the interrelations between the different actors in a global marketplace are complex and cannot be understood merely in terms of exclusion and repression. Apart from the generation of neo-colonial-like power relations the search for commercially valuable biogenetic or biochemical resources also includes the generation of an "ethics of sustainable development" and a fragmentation of sovereignty. From the beginning of the 1990s onwards, the assignment of economic value to biological resources has come to be seen as prerequisite for effective biodiversity conservation. In deed, an ethics of biodiversity conservation through assignment of economic value to plants is as old as the idea of bio- or chemical prospecting itself. From this perspective, potential profit extracted from the commercialization of rare species to be encountered in resource rich countries provides an incentive to halt the destruction of their natural habitats. Resource providers also started to struggle for shares in revenues gained by multinational corporations based on local knowledge about plants. In this context, fair bioprospecting was envisaged as a tool for sustainable development and community participation (Reid et al. 1993). The International Undertaking on Plant Genetic Resources that formerly declared biodiversity to be the common heritage of human kind was abandoned with the introduction of the UN Convention on Biological Diversity.

It is well know that CBD grants nation states autonomous rights over genetic resources on their territory and recognizes collective rights of indigenous communities, which must be protected by so called Access and Benefit-Sharing (ABS) agreements. Local stakeholders of a certain resource have to be informed about bioprospecting activities, must give their formal consent to it and have to be compensated if future revenues are to be achieved (Art. 8, 16, 19). In turn, local resource providers have to commit themselves to biodiversity conservation. In South Africa this framework was finally adopted by the implementation of the National Environmental Management Biodiversity Act. Applicants for patents must specify if their inventions are derived from indigenous biological resources or traditional use, which means the way in which or the purpose for which an indigenous community uses the resource in question. Subsequently, fair public-private partnerships between communities, state research institutions and pharmaceutical companies are envisioned.

There have been calls to reconsider market-oriented conservation in South Africa despite negative evidence from abroad. In terms of biodiversity, the country is still one of the richest on earth. However, due to the rising demand for medical plants and the shrinkage of habitats, many species are already facing local extinction. It is assumed that almost all medical plants available in urban markets in South Africa are harvested directly in their natural habitat, mostly in an unsustainable manner. In order to enhance biodiversity conservation, some ecologists are calling for large scale cultivation programs. Regionally there seems to be a growing harvesting pressure to meet the demand in metropolitan centers. Several authors call for an overall cooperation in conservation strategies considering the socio-economic realities of local consumers of these medicines and those who depend on the *muthi* trade for their livelihoods. Associated with the new interest in medicinal plants is not only an ethics of biodiversity conservation, but also an ethics of development similarly linked to the assignment of monetary value. It seems that the development of herbal medicines for regionally prevalent diseases is less relevant for such assignment.

The MRC with its program on traditional medicines against Malaria, Tuberculosis and AIDS-related infections still draws relatively little attention from potential private investors. There is however considerable interest in drugs that target North American and European life-style diseases. The Council for Scientific and Industrial Research has been successful in attracting several companies for the development of an appetite suppressant derived from the Hoodia cactus also used by the Khoisan. In 1995, the active substance named P57 encountered in the plant was patented by the CSIR. Six years later, a license to exploit the patent was granted to the UK based company Phytopharm. At the same time the San represented by the Working Group of Indigenous Minorities in Southern Africa (WIMSA), the South African San Council, and the San Institute of South Africa (SASI) claimed San ownership to the medicine.

The NGOs constructed a body of delegates that represented the San "community" and promoted negotiations with the CSIR. In 2003, the parties signed a benefit-sharing agreement that grants the CSIR and its partners the exclusive right to exploit the patent but enables the San to receive a six per cent share of the financial benefits received by the research institution from its private partners. In the case of success, approximately 0.03 percent to 1.2 percent of net sales of the product are entering a trust fund shared among the San Councils of Namibia, Botswana and South Africa.

The drug is currently in its last phase of clinical trials before being eventually distributed as a food supplement by the UK based multinational Unilever. Rachel Wynberg, board member of the Cape Town-based NGO Biowatch conceives the ABS agreement as a "historical breakthrough" although "there is a need for a more holistic, innovative and ethical approach to biodiversity commercialization beyond the models currently touted".

It has been claimed that unbalanced power relations between holders of local knowledge about *muthi* and scientists must be overcome to contribute to real social innovation through bioprospecting in South Africa.

From this perspective, effectiveness will depend as much on a more equitable "inward stretch" to endogenous knowledge as on "outward reach" to global sources. Until recently, the testing of biological activity of crude extracts and the isolation of compounds received much more attention than the interaction between plants and people, folk taxonomies, plant-related mythology, and pre-colonial plant use. The extent to which an ethics based on market-principles in Post-Apartheid South Africa is able to bridge the gap between different values accorded to medicinal plants is far from being evident yet.

CONCLUSION

The process of bioprospecting involves a double translation of knowledge from traditional healers about plant based medicines and spells (*muthi*) into patentable scientific knowledge about chemical compounds and back again in terms of new property regimes introduced through Access and Benefit-Sharing (ABS) agreements.

In this process, herbal medicine becomes an asset which is manipulated and transformed in relation to its capacity to promote health, its market value, and its potential to construct a new ethics of development. Property rights on *muthi* become transformed through local communities, state, and corporate interests and, on the other hand, also generate new institutions, alliances and discourses.

The above mentioned examples indicate a synchronicity of the exploitation of local medical resources based on clear-cut sovereign power relations and more flexible ones in which actors and institutions of different social, ethnic and organizational strata are aligned in the same network of mutual interest.

Traditional healers and San communities challenge their share in the economy of values and adopt new property regimes on their own. However, under the label of empowerment and participation which adds ethical value to state institutions and multinational corporations, still lurk historic power differentials between North and South as well as between scientists, holders of local knowledge and resource providers.

In the alignment of actors and actants, the South African state still holds a hegemonic position and is drawn between the revitalization of TM as part of an identity politics that makes up for the impudence towards local knowledge in the past, on the one hand, and the interest in marketable culture on the other.

The World Trade Organization (WTO) and the Agreement on Trade Related Aspects of Intellectual Property Rights (TRIPS) do not recognize collective rights based on culture. While this is inconsistent with the CBD, currently, still surprisingly little is known about how rights of ownership and control of IK are actually negotiated in everyday transactions between scientists, pharmaceutical companies, traditional healers and local communities.

By following a particular *muthi* and its plant ingredients from specific rural collection or cultivation sites to the laboratory and back again, ethnographic studies would be able to identify how, in actuality, value is conceptualized among the different stakeholders, how rights to ownership are negotiated between them and what consequences this has for the promotion of a more equitable sharing of power and knowledge in the proclaimed African Renaissance. Such an analysis would certainly start with an emic view on regimes of value among plant collectors and petty traders. Given that existing studies show that women are primarily involved in plant harvesting in rural areas, it is important to disclose how gender relations relate to the "hidden" *muthi* economy. Whether evolving cultivation projects challenge the economic survival of low income women and their families or if they have a positive impact on poverty reduction remains to be seen.

Several Anthropologists pointed out that the attempt to copyright culture by particular fractions or organizations at the expense of others might contribute to the schism of communities and fuel the establishment of ethnic boundaries. The granting of rights on the basis of ethnicity uncomfortably reminds us of Apartheid ideology.

In fact, the well-intentioned benefit-sharing efforts promoted by the CBD depict a static and essential image of local culture by assuming bluntly that neo-liberal property regimes could be applied universally. While the convention addresses the misappropriation of local knowledge, it also generates new power differentials. Local medical knowledge cannot be confined to clear-cut ethnic boundaries due to well-documented dynamics of diffusion and exchange between different identity groups.

To date it is not quite clear if the establishment of "trust funds" will ban such dynamics. It will be of special interest to document how far ABS agreements are contributing to a revitalized codification of local knowledge alongside ethnic boundaries and/ or in relation to different types of healers and their adjunct organizations.

Since there are no frameworks for assuring the representativeness of healers or other stakeholders in negotiations and ABS agreements, there is also great potential for conflict between the included and the excluded parties. The discrimination between *inyangas* in terms of pure herbalists and *sangomas* in terms of spiritual practitioners may contribute to rivalries as the latter become excluded from evolving power/knowledge networks. Future research will have to pay special attention to their strategies and tactics to enclose and protect knowledge. Indeed, it is hardly known how far bioprospecting in South Africa requires healers and local plant providers to re-conceptualize values accorded to medicinal plants, particularly in the face of new property rights.

Apart from concerns with the knowledge creation process underlying patenting, it becomes increasingly important to address the ethical dimension of separating biochemically relevant information from *muthi* and the context in which it is entwined. Biovalue can only be assigned through translation, which involves the transformation of *muthi* to standardized scientific knowledge capable of being turned into intellectual property. It still remains to be addressed how value regimes, tied to locally situated social and cultural actors and actants that come with the substance(s), are concealed step by step through technology. Anthropological studies on bioprospecting in South Africa will have to consider the entanglement of the very scientific research institutions in particular cultures and societies.

The institutions involved in bioprospecting are about to transform organizational structures and processes in accordance with the values assigned to the subject of study. This is likely to transform knowledge production and reproduction itself. One of the biggest challenges in this respect will be to analyze how market-oriented research transforms the very sciences of ethnobotany, ethnobiology and ethnopharmacology.

How do scientists themselves mediate their new role as businessmen, on the one hand, and as ethical arbitrators in access and benefit-sharing endeavors on the other? What impact has the search for commercially valuable and ethically appropriated resources on the topics chosen or the findings obtained in the laboratory? Finally, the problem of how to share, with whom and on what basis may turn into a matter of informal decision-making based on an ethics directed by the neo-liberal market.

The extent to which the transformation of regimes of value on medicinal plants promotes, facilitates or prohibits an African Renaissance remains to be seen. One of the myths generated in its context is the value accorded to bioprospecting as technique to simultaneously enhance the health of the 'previously' disadvantaged, to reduce poverty, to help develop a "positive" African identity, and to protect the natural environment. While there are indicators for its failure, these will have to be addressed more thoroughly by empirical research to come. Ten years after the announcement of the new nation-building project the (bio)prospect for a renaissance through so-called Traditional Medicine has neither met the high expectations of its supporters nor entailed the devastating effects of its opponents.

7

Medicinal Plants Used by the Yi Ethnic Group

BACKGROUND

Study Area

Chuxiong Prefecture, located in the north of middle Yunnan Plateau (24°13' – 26°30' N, 100°43' – 102°43' E), has numerous high mountains, deep canyons, and large and small rivers. Mountainous land in Chuxiong occupies over 90% of its total territory. Chuxiong's climate is considered a sub-tropical and moist plateau monsoon climate, primarily affected by two air currents: a warm, dry current from northern Africa, the Middle-East and the subcontinent of India during winter and a cool, moist current from the Indian Ocean and Bay of Bengal during summer. The climate of Chuxiong is characterized by long spring and autumn and short summer and winter. Although the daily temperature can vary greatly, the climate is generally temperate and without extremes. The Ailao Mountains contain large forests and are abundant with medicinal plants. The Yi have utilized these plants in the prevention and cure of disease for centuries. Some 871 species of Yi plant medicines have currently been recorded.

Population

With the exception of the Han Chinese, there are 55 minority nationalities in China. Each of them has their own unique history and medicinal system. With a population of 6.57 million, the Yi are the sixth largest minority in China, distributed in Yunnan, Sichuan, Guizhou and Guangxi provinces. In the southwest of China, Yunnan holds the largest population of the Yi nationality, which reaches 4.06 million.

Aim of study

Research into the literature reveals that most of the ancient books on Yi medicine were handed down by dictation and are hand-written. Therefore, there must be additional traditional knowledge on Yi medicine that was scattered among folk areas and unrecorded, including some proven remedies with special curative effects preserved by folk doctors. We thus decided to collect the folk knowledge of Yi medicine in Chuxiong Prefecture to compliment the previously documented works on traditional Yi medicine.

PREVIOUS KNOWLEDGE ON LOCAL FOLK MEDICINE

The Yi people mainly inhabit mountainous areas or river valleys. The particular geology and climate is ideal for a unique Yi medicine effective in treating pyretic toxicity, rheumatics, etc. Yi medicine, practiced for 3000 years, is derived from Dali medicine of the Nanshao Kingdom. By assimilating the best of local, Indian, and Persian medicine, the Yi people built their own medicinal theoretical system. The Yi acquired extensive clinical experience and recorded the pertinent knowledge in books, such as *Xian Yao Jing*, *Shuangbai Medicinal Book of Yi Nationality*, *Book for Curing Diseases*, and others. The earliest book of Yi medicine is *The Shuangbai Medicinal Book of Yi Nationality*, written even earlier than Shi-Zhen Li's *Ben Cao Gang Mu* in 1758.

As we know, traditional medicine (TM) is widely used and is of increasing importance in a rapidly growing global health and economic system. In Africa, up to 80% of the population uses TM to help to meet their health care needs. In Asia and South America, populations continue to use TM as a result of historical circumstances and cultural beliefs. In China, TM accounts for around 40% of all health care delivered.

Given these statistics, we should cherish, protect and develop upon the legacy that is traditional Yi medicine.

The majority of products which were exploited in recent years based on Yi medicines have provided positive social and financial benefits. The famous Yi doctor, Huan-Zhang Qu, researched and developed the outstanding *Yunnan Bai Medicine*. Similar drugs such as the *Capsule of Paiduyangyan*, the *Kunming Shanhaitang*, the *Injection of Yunnan Dengzhanhua*, *Injection of Sanqi saponin*, *Capsule of Yixinkang* and others have all been developed following deep research into the culture of traditional Yi medicine. The selling price of these drugs derived from traditional Yi medicines could reach 10 billion Chinese Yuan (or 1.26 billions in US dollars) per year.

Indigenous knowledge, and folk knowledge in particular, continues to be impacted by mainstream culture and decreasing biodiversity; traditional practices using specific medicinal plants decreases more quickly than that of the general biodiversity. It is thus urgent and necessary to prevent the further loss of the specialized knowledge of minority peoples. This is best accomplished by gathering and documenting their unique practices and their relationships to medicinal plants.

Methodology

Eight field surveys in four counties were carried out during different seasons over a period of four years (1999–2002). These four locations in Chuxiong Prefecture consisted of: Wuding, Shuangbai and Nanhua counties, and Chuxiong City. The methodological approaches were used in ethnobotany, anthropology, and participatory rural appraisal (PRA) were adopted for the field investigations.

During each visit, detailed field records were taken on the functions of plants and the plant parts that were used. Information was obtained through interviews with 32 informants including elderly villagers, local healers, and herbalists. The authors collected voucher specimens of 116 plants in the field with assistance from local herbalists. The specimens were later verified using *The Flora of China* and *Illustrated Handbook for Higher Plants of China*, and by the authors, plant taxonomists, and experts from the authors' institution. The voucher specimens were deposited in the Voucher Herbarium of the Laboratory of Ethnobotany, Kunming Institute of Botany, Chinese Academy of Sciences. The local names of the herbs, their life forms, preparation methods, and their useful parts for treating various diseases were carefully recorded in the field. The efficacy of these plants was also analyzed and compared with the pertinent literature.

RESULTS

Statistics of Plants Used

One hundred and sixteen plant species used for medicinal purposes by people living in Chuxiong Prefecture of Yunnan Province were collected and identified. These species are represented by 58 different families, of which Compositae (15 species), Rosaceae (6 species), and Liliaceae, Papilionaceae and Orchidaceae (each with 5 species) hold the highest number of species used medicinally. One hundred and four genera are represented: *Ainsliaea*, *Artemisia*, *Clematis*, *Clerodendrum*, *Conyza*, *Corydalis*, *Cynanchum*, *Indigofera*, *Pholidota*, *Polygala*, *Polygonum* and *Rubus* all occurring twice.

25 previously unidentified species (21.55%) were found to have new curative effects and 40 species (34.48%) had preparation methods that have never been recorded in the contemporary medical texts of the Yi nationality in Chuxiong Prefecture.

Medicinal Uses

The three most common conditions treated with Yi plants were: trauma, such as wounds and fractures, for which 55 different species were used, eg. *Crepis napifera* and *Gaultheria yunnanensis*; gastrointestinal disorders, such as stomachache, diarrhea, and constipation; and the common cold, such as fever, cough, sore throat and influenza (for example, *Murraya paniculata* and *Polygonum cymosum*). Only nine species were reported as being useful against a single disease, eg. *Ranunculus ternatus* and *Euonymus japonicus*.

Table 1. List of the frequency of ailments treated with medicinal plants

Disease	Species used	% of total
Trauma	55	47.41%
Gastrointestinal disorders	47	40.52%
Common cold	24	20.69%
Skin problems	20	17.24%
Liver problems	19	16.38%
Gynaecopathia	18	15.52%
Inflammation	13	11.21%
Trachea/bronchi disorder	12	10.34%
Edema	11	9.48%
Lung problems	11	9.48%
Antitoxics	10	8.62%
Heart problems	10	8.62%
Body pains	9	7.76%
Female issues	5	4.31%
Blood problems	4	3.45%
Eye problems	4	3.45%
Kidney problems	4	3.45%
Neural diseases	3	2.59%
Cypridopathy	2	1.72%
Ear problems	2	1.72%
Mouth cavity problems	2	1.72%
Infectious disease	1	0.86%
Parasitic diseases	1	0.86%
Rhachitis	1	0.86%
Tooth problems	1	0.86%

PLANT HABIT AND PART USED

Seventy two plants, over half of the species used medicinally, were herbaceous in nature (eg. *Ainsliaea yunnanensis* and *Cucubalus baccifer*), while 33 were woody, i.e. tree, shrub, or woody liana (eg. *Aquilaria sinensis* and *Toona sinensis*), and 11 were sub-shrubs. The entire plant was used most often, accounting for 65 species out of 116 (56.03%), followed by the roots, of 42 species out of 116 (36.21%); other plant parts were used less frequently, about 7.76%.

PREPARING METHODS OF MEDICINAL PLANTS

The preparing methods of medicinal plants were different and special. Eighty-eight species could be taken by decoction, which was the most common preparing method. Seventeen species should be used after they were soaking in alcohol. Four species could be used after making juice for drinking or external uses. Fourteen species could be used by making powder. Some species should be used together with other species, or with sugar, honey, meat, eggs, chicken, or other materials.

CONCLUSION

In the present study, 116 species belonging to 58 families have been identified as medicinal plants used by Yi healers in Chuxiong Prefecture, Yunnan Province. These plants have unique properties and are used in the treatment of trauma, gastrointestinal disorders and the common cold. From the statistic data, we found most of the plants are used to treat trauma. This is because the primitive ancestors of the Yi people usually lived in tree crotches and made their living by hunting and gathering, which made them vulnerable to injury. The medicinal plants used to treat gastrointestinal disorders accounts for the second largest percentage. This result can be explained by the epidemiological research on *Helicobacter pylori* (Hp) among Yi communities. The Yi people were easily infected by Hp, which has a strong correlation with their fondness for drinking distilled spirits, smoking, and eating pickled, fermented, and fried food.

There are several characteristics of traditional Yi medicine. Most plants used in Yi medicine are herbaceous. Among 116 medicinal plant species traditionally used by the Yi healers in the case sites, 72 species are either perennial or annual herbs, or herbaceous lianas. This is partially due to the Yi's polytheistic beliefs. The Yi believe that both mountains and big trees are sacred and should not be harmed. This perception of nature plays a positive role on the protection of the vegetation around their dwelling places. The minorities who live in mountainous areas would never intentionally damage their natural environment and aim to exist in harmony with it. That is why many scholars advocate that people living in modern society learn from the minority people, to respect the environment rather than depredating it. Fresh herbs are used almost exclusively by Yi healers. Dry herbs are used, but much less frequently. The Yi healers usually used a single herb instead of multi-species compounds. For example, when the Yi healer treated wounds with *Gaultheria yunnanensis*, he would not mix it with any of the other (over 50) species he knew that could also treat wounds. Some healers were less concerned about measuring doses when administering medicinal herbs. Medicinal plant preparation methods vary: For external application, plants are generally pounded, kneaded or chewed; for oral doses, plants are often chewed, decocted or cooked with meat.

Traditional Yi medicine is especially characterized by its use of alcohol. The Yi people adore alcohol, and it has come to symbolically represent this cultural minority due to its significance in their lives. Home-made alcohol is the most important beverage for the Yi: it is used daily, for ceremonies and holidays, served to respected guests and friends, and is the most common method of administering plant medicines. The practice of combining plants and alcohol has a long history in Yi medicine. Yi healers use different procedures to administer their raw material/alcohol combinations. They most commonly use:

(1) Medicinal alcohol: medicinal plants and/or animals are soaked in alcohol for about a month and the resulting liquid then is drunk by the patient or applied externally to the affected parts;

(2) Alcohol decoction: herbs are put into alcohol, decocted and drunk;

(3) Alcohol as solvent instead of water: fresh plant liquid or dried plant powder is placed in alcohol and either drunk or applied externally; and

(4) Burning alcohol in medicine: medicinal plants are mixed with alcohol, heated, and then either taken by mouth or applied externally.

It is believed that alcohol extracts more active components from the medicinal plants than water does, thus being more effective in curing diseases. For example, *Ainsliaea latifolia* var. *obovata*, when soaked in alcohol, is far more effective in treating children's fever than the fresh plant alone. This traditional knowledge was previously unreported.

Since natural medicines can cure diseases ranging from bacterial infections to cancers, pharmaceutical companies and the public recognize the importance of its development. Most of the pharmaceutical companies believe that the biggest benefit hiding behind the traditional plant knowledge and practices of minority people is the value of new drug development.

Biodiversity is a rare gift provided by nature to those researching chemo-diversity and the discovery of new drugs. This chemo diversity not only provides the necessary secondary metabolites of plant evolution, but also provides abundant lead compounds, the basis of new drug development. Due to the side-effects associated with chemosynthetic medicine and environmental pollution, medical scientists from both here and abroad have begun to look into the realm of traditional medicine, which has used natural medicine as its main remedial measure. During our research, we found twenty five species with previously undocumented curative effects and forty species whose preparation methods and compatibilities had not been documented. These new records can be an important source for further phytochemical, pharmacological and clinical studies.

8

Valorizing the 'Irulas' Traditional Knowledge of Medicinal Plants

A mounting body of critical research is raising the credibility of Traditional Knowledge (TK) in scientific studies. These studies have gained credibility because their claims are supported by methods that are repeatable and provide data for quantitative analyses that can be used to assess confidence in the results. The theoretical importance of our study is to test consensus (reliability/replicable) of TK within one ancient culture; the Irulas of the Kodiakkarai Reserve Forest (KRF), India. We calculated relative frequency (RF) and consensus factor (F_{ic}) of TK from 120 Irulas informants knowledgeable of medicinal plants. Our research indicates a high consensus of the Irulas TK concerning medicinal plants.

The Irulas revealed a diversity of plants that have medicinal and nutritional utility in their culture and specific ethnotaxa used to treat a variety of illnesses and promote general good health in their communities. Throughout history aboriginal people have been the custodians of bio-diversity and have sustained healthy life-styles in an environmentally sustainable manner. However this knowledge has not been transferred to modern society. We suggest this may be due to the asymmetry between scientific and TK, which demands a new approach that considers the assemblage of TK and scientific knowledge. A greater understanding of TK is beginning to emerge based on our research with both the Irulas and Malasars; they believe that a healthy lifestyle is founded on a healthy environment. These aboriginal groups chose to share this knowledge with society-at-large in order to promote a global lifestyle of health and environmental sustainability.

BACKGROUND

A mounting body of critical research is raising the credibility of Traditional Knowledge (TK) in scientific studies and natural resource management. The lack of recognition of the place and value TK in science has prevented real engagement of this knowledge in scientific endeavours including nutrition, medicine, environmental assessment and resource management practices. One explanation is the lack of validation using quantitative analyses that give some measure of confidence and methods for replication. Clearly there is some asymmetry between scientific and TK, which requires new approaches to the relationship between scientific and TK. We must consider some criteria for negotiating and legitimating the validity of knowledge. Science is based on the evolution of knowledge, which is testable and ultimately generalisable, mobile and globally meaningful.

To gain credibility, scientific studies that utilize TK must be reliable (refutable) and designed so that they can be replicated. The need for full disclosure in science demands quantitative measures of the reliability to be established. In ethnobotanical studies, this was established by Trotter and Logan who developed a quantitative method to evaluate consensus among informants in order to identifying potentially effective medicinal plants. Consensus analysis provides a measure of reliability for any given claim providing refutable evidence. This evolved into the "Factor of informant Consensus" (FIC) in order to quantitatively evaluate the degree of selection of certain plants for a particular utility (e.g, healing an ailment). One of the traditional intentions of FIC is to test the homogeneity among informants' knowledge. Researchers use consensus analysis to test falsifiable hypotheses concerning informant selection and use of plants, as a decision making factor, to weight the relative importance of TK, and to estimate the competence of informants. These studies have gained credibility because their claims are supported by methods that are repeatable and provide data for quantitative analyses that can be used to assess confidence in the results.

India is rich in ethnic diversity and traditional knowledge (TK) that has resulted in a considerable body of ethnobotanical research, of which one study has revealed a deep understanding of medicinal plants supported by high consensus. There are over 537 different aboriginal groups in India with extensive knowledge of plants. Many qualitative surveys have recorded detailed utility of specific plants for many aboriginal groups such as the Malasars, Malamalasars, Malayalis, Irulas, Gonds, Koysd, Konda reddis, Valmikis, Koyas, Chenchus, Lambadis, Jatapus, Savaras, Bagatas, Kammaras, Khondas, Nukadoras, Porjas, Jatapus, Paliyar, Kanikar, Todas, Kotas, Kattunayakas, Apatani and Chellipale. Recent research by Ragupathy et al. presented the first quantitative research in India that considers variation in TK among informants using a quantitative consensus analysis. Their research discovered high consensus in TK and new insights in medicinal utility by the Malasars towards understanding their vital well being and good health. This research provided several alternative hypotheses for consensus of TK that may be low when considering different spatial scales, unreliable TK, informant bias, localized remedies, variability in local ethnotaxa, availability of multiple traditional remedies or recent replacement by pharmaceutical supplements.

The theoretical importance of our study is to test consensus (reliability/replicable) of TK within one ancient culture; the Irulas of the Kodiakkarai Reserve Forest (KRF) in the Coromandal coast of Thanjavur district, India. We chose to work with the Irulas of India, because they are known to be exceptional healers and keepers of TK of the flora in the coastal forest and there is limited research on the Irula's TK. Furthermore, the Irulas are an example of a culture that has preserved a highly diverse area ecosystem that sustains their healthy life-styles. We hypothesize that consensus of TK of specific plants used for different illness categories are high indicating reliable TK among informants at a local scale (within one localized aboriginal group or community – Irulas of the KRF), because it has been used within their culture without interruption for many generations. This hypothesis concurs with the results of our study of the Malasars TK of medicinal plants. Scientific inquiry demands that research can be replicated in order to substantiate claims of medicinal utility within any aboriginal culture.

Alternatively, consensus of TK may be low at local scales because of (i) unreliable TAK, (ii) informant bias, (iii) local remedies; certain villages may have unique uses for plants, (iv) variability in local ethnotaxa; certain communities may have found variants or ecotypes for some plants that result in unique qualities that are of particular use at only a local scale, (v) use of pharmaceutical supplements; the availability of modern pharmaceuticals for a particular ailment may result sporadic use of traditional remedies, and (vi) availability of multiple remedies; there may be groups of plants and therefore several remedies available that are preferentially selected by individual healers for various utilities (e.g, healing some ailment), thus indicating the potential biological activity for a group of plants. These groups may represent Linnaean taxa (i.e, genus or family) that share similar biological processes, or aboriginal classifications may group plants that serve a similar utility.

THE IRULAS AND THEIR LAND – ETHNOGRAPHY

The Irulas are as small tribal community that is part of the Dravidian language group that is spoken in south-eastern India. They are recognized as a Scheduled Tribe (ST) by the Government of India. Most ethnic populations of southern India are linguistically Dravidian. The Irulas belong to the Negrito (or Negroid) race, which is one of the six main ethnic groups that add to the racial mosaic of India. Negroids from Africa were the oldest people to have migrated to India. The structure of their tribal dialects is slightly different from modern Dravidians. The Dravidians of South India speak Tamil, Telugu and Malyalam, but the Irulas in KRF speak a different dialect of Tamil, which is distantly related to other

Dravidian Tamil. The Irulas, the largest Tamil speaking adivasi (Aboriginal) tribe in Tamil Nadu, found themselves virtually bonded labourers in 1976 when the Forest Protection Bill deprived many of their traditional lifestyle. The Irulas started moving to the neighbouring villages in hope of rebuilding their lives. The origin of the word "Irulas" is not clear. Some surmise that it is derived from the Tamil word, 'Irul', implying the dark complexion of the Irulas often being spotted by villagers as distant silhouettes in the forests, and supporting their local name, "the Forest People".

The culture of the Irulas has changed little over the last thousand years. Their staple food consists of minor millets, grain legumes, and wild yams supplemented with rice. They do not practice agriculture and therefore wholly depend on forest produce and wild animals like wild bore, rabbit, rat, deer, wildcat and fish. The Irulas settlements are located within or on the edge of the forests and consist of tiny scattered huts. The community is divided into several exogamous clans. Marriage between inhabitants of different hamlets is generally encouraged and patrilocal residence is commonplace. More recently, some Irulas go to local villages to trade or sell honey, honey wax, firewood, wild fruits, yams, wild Carissa, Manilkara and Solanum berries and other native herbal products. This supports a productive and localized non-timber forest product (NTFP) industry, which supports many families. The Irulas trade NTFPs for local farm produce such as rice, potato, eggplant, tomato, tea, cookies and spices. Other occupations of the Irulas include intermittent farm labour and the legendary profession of snake charming. They have distinct cultural and religious practices, including worship of the Goddess Kanniamma, and appointment of Pujari 'priests' to serve their communities.

Biogeography of the Study Site

Kodiakkarai Reserve Forest (KRF) is a dry evergreen tropical forest located on the Coromandel Coast of Thanjavur district, Tamil Nadu, South India, 325 km south of Madras city, the capital of Tamil Nadu. The reserve covers an area of about 25 sq. km.

Geographically the KRF lies at latitude 10° 18' N and longitude 79° 51' E, and is bordered by the Bay of Bengal to the east and Palk Strait to the south. The elevation ranges 25 to 50 m above mean sea level. Like most other costal areas in Thanjavur District, the climate of KRF is warm and moist. Monthly mean temperature of the area is between 24°C and 32°C, with maximum temperatures rising to 41°C and minimum temperatures near 29°C. Monthly mean percentage of humidity is between 60% and 80%, with a maximum of 92.3% during October and a minimum of 69.6% in April. The annual precipitation ranges from 1000 – 1500 mm with the wet South West monsoon occurring from June until September. The KRF is often impacted by serious erosion during the Southwest monsoon because of the heavy rainfall in the Western Ghats washes loose soil from the hills that invariably feeds the Cauvery River and empties into the Indian Ocean.

The diversity of wildlife in the KRF is rich and includes many tropical species of monkeys, jackals and foxes. The coastal belt of dry evergreen forest at Kodiakkarai hosts large populations of spotted deer, antelopes and wild pigs. Crocodiles once existed in large numbers but they have now dwindled due to over-hunting. The swamps of Point Calimere within the KRF contain over 240 bird species, including large populations of flamingos and a rich diversity of stints, ducks, herons, painted storks, teals, terns, pelicans, egrets, sand pipers and Mongolian plovers. The plant diversity includes more than 370 species of vascular plants within three main floristic regions: dry evergreen forest, wet forests (mangroves) and grasslands.

METHODS

Ethnobotanical Survey and Consensus Analysis

Our survey protocols are identical to our previous study of the Malasars in the Velliangiri Hills of India. These methods follow standard methods for interviews, data confirmation and field observation as suggested by Bernard; Etkin; Pelto and Pelto; Alexiades. To elucidate community domains and determine differences in TK among the informants we cross checked with new informants to determine the percent frequency of a particular response within our survey. The local 'headman' helped to us record general information on the local customs, habits and beliefs, information on the surrounding area and individuals who are knowledgeable of the local flora and could serve as informants.

The consensus analysis utilized the informant's TK as defined by the surveys. Local informants (i.e., traditional healers) having practical knowledge of plant medicinal utility of the KRF were interviewed during April 2005 – January 2007. During the course of the study, about 7 field trips were conducted in the study area. Surveys were conducted by a stratified random selection of informants, based on methods suggested by Schultes, Jain and Bernard. Successive free listing was used to interview 100 informants providing data for the consensus analysis. The informants were selected following standard interview protocols. We interviewed over 120 informants from which we selected 80 informants that were equally distributed among four different age categories; elders, middle aged, teenagers, < 10 years.

During these interviews we documented all possible information about a specific plant and then sorted this information according to utilitarian perspective, local name or ecology. The informants were given limited time and there was no differentiation among gender. We also asked the informants to group the plant specimens into different illness categories that were predefined from previous research, and through consultation with the headman and individual informants. We requested all informants to collect specimens of the common plants they knew or to show the plant species on site. The questionnaires were used to obtain information on medicinal plants with their local names, parts used, mode of preparation and administration.

The relative frequency (RF) of TK from each individual ethnotaxa from the interviews was calculated to determine a quantitative value for validating TK of ethnotaxa utility (eg, remedy of choice). Although being named by three informants is the most common cut-off point to establish consensus, we choose to calculate the RF for all TK with respect to each ethnotaxa. Calculation of a consensus factor (F_{ic}) for testing homogeneity of informant's knowledge followed methods of Trotter and Logan. A consensus factor of F_{ic} is given by:

$$F_{ic} = Nur - Nt/(Nur - 1).$$

The factor provides a range of 0 to 1, where a high value acts as a good indicator for a high rate of informant consensus. Nur is the number of use-reports of informants for particular illness usage, where a use-report is a single record for use of a plant mentioned by an individual, and Nt refers to the number of species used for a particular illness category for all informants. The majority of illness types are grouped into predefined ethno/economic botany categories, with the additions of a few other illness categories that were commonly mentioned during our interviews because they were prevalent in these communities. The use of "general categories" is adopted here as recommended by other ethnobotanical researchers. These 30 illnesses were sorted into 12 usage categories. All of the illness types were translated as best as possible from the Irulas description of the illness/symptoms to known biomedical terms, with few exceptions (e.g., spiritualism – keep family wellness/repel evil).

Table: Irulas ailments grouped by illness category

Illness Category	**Biomedical/English Term**	**Irulas Term**
Dermatological	Skin disease	*Thol viyathi*
	Skin appearance	*Palapalappu*
Diabetes	Diabetes	*Chakari noie*
Fever	Fever	*Kaichal*
Gastrointestinal	Diarrhoea	*Vaitru po'kku*
	Purgative	*Vaitru po'kku*
	Intestinal worms	*Vaitru poochi*
General health	Complementary food	*Siru ounavu*
	Antidotes	*Visha murichi*
	Anti mosquito	*Nochi vadai*

	General medicine	*Podhu maruthuvam*
	Cold	*Shzali*
	Antibiotic	*Ethir nachu*
	Lethargy	*Kayakalpa*
	Appetite	*Pasi edupu*
	Hypothermia	*Soodu thanippu*
	Blood Flow	*Ratha o'ttam*
Hydrocele	Hydrocele	*Virai veengi*
Infection	Wounds	*Kayam*
Jaundice	Jaundice	*Manjal kamalai*
Leprosy	Leprosy	*Thozhu noie*
Pain	Headache	*Thalai vali*
	Eye pain	*Kan vali*
	Earache	*Kadhu vali*
	Toothache	*Pal vali*
	Pregnancy pain	*Prasava vali*
	Body ache	*Udambu vali*
	Rheumatism	*Moottu vadham*
Respiratory	Asthma	*Izhuppu*
	Cough	*Irummal*
Spiritual	Wellness	

BOTANICAL DOCUMENTATION AND PRESERVATION

All plants utilized in the interviews were collected as vouchers for confirmation of identity using the Irulas classification system. The Linnaean identities were designated by comparing the specimens with the authentic type specimens in herbaria, and by referring to recent taxonomic monographs and revisions.

The botanical nomenclature followed that of Flora of Tamil Nadu, India Series I Analysis. Live species were propagated and can be found in the E.K. Janakiammal Etnobotanical Garden, Botany Field Research Laboratory, University of Madras, Maduravoyal,

Chennai. Voucher specimens are deposited in the herbarium of the University of Madras, Chennai, and the herbarium of Botanical Survey of India, Southern Circle (MH).

RESULTS AND DISCUSSION

Consensus of the Irulas TK of Medicinal Plants

Our research indicates a high level of consensus of TK of medicinal plants within the Irulas community. In our study, the relative frequency (RF) of TK from each individual ethnotaxa from the interviews was high (mean RF = 0.92 ± 0.04).

The informant consensus of medicinal plant usage resulted in F_{ic} ranging from 0.70 to 1.00 per illness category. The average F_{ic} value for all illness categories was 0.85, indicating a high level of informant consensus compared to similar studies from other countries.

In the literature, high informant consensus was also recorded among studies with many illness categories such as a study with the Malasars (F_{ic} = 0.71) in India and several studies focused on specific illness categories: the snakebite healers of Kamba in Africa (F_{ic} = 0.88); and treating 'mich' or febrile diseases (F_{ic} = 0.80), and respiratory disorders (F_{ic} = 0.88) among Inuit in Nunavut.

We recently publishedthe first study to utilize a consensus analysis in ethnobotanical research within India. This research investigated the Malasars occupying the forests of the Velliangiri holy hills in the Western Ghats, South India.

The results of this research revealed 95 ethnotaxa that are utilized by the Malasars for medicinal and general health purposes of which most had high consensus (F_{ic} > 0.80) for some ailments such as respiratory and jaundice.

Our current research is exploring the consensus of TK with respect to the same ethnotaxa across spatial (beyond local geographic villages) and cultural scales (among different cultures such as the Irulas and Malasars).

Table: Ethnobotanical consensus index for traditional medicinal plant use categories

Illness category	Number of use-reports (N_{ur})	Number of Taxa (N_t)	Informants' consensus index factor (F_{ic})[a]
Dermatological	12	3	0.82
Diabetes	7	1	1.00
Fever	12	4	0.73
Gastrointestinal	17	5	0.75
General health	61	19	0.70
Hydorcoele	6	1	1.00
Infection	13	4	0.75
Jaundice	6	1	1.00
Leprosy	5	1	1.00
Pain	46	14	0.71
Respiratory	8	2	0.86
Spiritual	13	2	0.92

[a]$F_{ic} = N_{ur}-N_t/(N_{ur}-1)$, providing a value between 0 and 1, where high value indicates a high rate of informant consensus.

DIVERSITY OF ETHNOTAXA UTILIZED BY THE IRULAS FOR MEDICINE

The Irulas revealed a diversity of plants that have medicinal and nutritional utility in their culture. During this study the Irulas informed us of 53 ethnotaxa that have considerable utility in medicinal and general health care purposes within their culture. This body of TK concerning medicinal and nutritional plants was supported by high consensus (mean $F_{ic} = 0.85 \pm 0.04$). We provide the medicinal utility and method of preparation for each ethnotaxa in Table below. The 53 common ethnotaxa were classified within Linnaean taxonomy to represent 52 species distributed in 51 genera belonging to 33 families of plants. The Irulas prefer to utilize species from primary or secondary dry evergreen coastal forests of Coromandal Coast of Thanjavur district, Southeast India, rather than the weedy species from disturbed areas.

Table 3. Irulas medicinal utility of the flora in the Kodiakarai Reserve Forest (KRF)

Botanical Name and Family	Tamil Lexicon	Method of Preparation and Medicinal Uses
Acanthaceae		
	Auduthoda	Extracts of root, bark, leaves, and flowers used for cough. Dried leaves emhaled for rapid recovery from asthma. Fresh flowers kept over the eyes to relieve eye pain.
Amaranthaceae		
Achyranthes aspera L.	*Nagarasi*	Extract of leaves along with palm jaggery fed to new born babies. Inflorescence scratched against mother breasts to increase lactation.
Aerva lanata (L.) Juss.ex Schult	*Celosia argentea* L.	*Kannupila & Pannaipoo* Whole plant harvested from the forest or sacred groves during festival day (Farmers Thanksgiving Day), which is used spiritually for healing sour necks of bull.
Aristolochiaceae		
Aristolochia indica L.	*Perumanthikodi*	Root tubers ground with a little water, mixed with rice or cow's milk to cure a fever.
Arecaceae		
Borassus flabellifer L.*Phoenix sylvestris* (L.) Roxb.	*PanaiInjai*	Toddy tapped from the inflorescence. Brushes and ropes prepared from leaf sheaths. Leaves used for thatching.Meristematic portion of the stem eaten by pregnant women from 9th month onwards for relief from abdominal pain.

Asclepiadaceae		
Gymnema sylvestre R.Br.	*Sirukurinjan & hakarikolli*	Tender fresh leaves and dried powder are used to cure diabetes. Cooked leaves may also be used in meals to treat diabetes.
Asteraceae		
Tridax procumbens L.	*Vettukayapoondu*	Leaf juice applied on wounds to stop bleeding.
Caparidaceae		
Capparis sepiaria L. *Capparis zeylanica* L.	*ThorattiAdandai*	Root pulp applied on small wounds and scratches.Leaves mixed with pepper, tamarind and garlic into a paste, which is consumed to increase appetite.
Cucurbitaceae		
Trichosanthes cucumerina L.	*Peyppadal*	Ripe fruit contains a mucilaginous exudate, which is applied directly on forehead to treat headaches.
Caesalpiniaceae		
Cassia auriculata L.	*Avarai*	The leaves, flowers, fruits, stems and roots are used to maintain hygiene of the skin and scalp. Every year, the first day of the month of crop harvest is celebrated as the thanks-giving day for the "bull".
Ebenaceae		
Diospyros ferrea (Wild.) Bahk. Var. *buxifolia*	*Veeraii*	Fruit improves blood circulation.

Euphorbiaceae		
Acalypha indica L.	*Kuppaimeni*	Decoction of leaves used for ear pain, snake bite and scabies.
Excoecaria agallocha L.	*Thillai*	Latex applied on wounds for antiseptic.
Jatropha tanjorensis Ellis & Saroja	*Katamanukku*	Latex heals wounds.
Phyllanthus amarus Schum. . & Thonn	*Kizhanelli*	Raw branchlets and leaves eaten for 7 days for curing jaundice.
Fabaceae		
Acacia nilotica (L.) Willd. ex. Del.	*Karuvelam*	Paste of tender leaves used to control dysentery. Gum powder mixed with the white of an egg, and applied on burns or scalds.
Albizia lebbeck (L.) Benth.	*Vagai*	Oil extracted from the seeds smeared on wounds for healing or on the lesions of lepers.
Caesalpinia bonduc (L.) Roxb.	*Kazhchikai*	Seeds are made into a paste to treat a hydrocele
Canavalia lineata (Thunb.) DC.	*Kozhiavarai*	Roasted seeds of *Mucuna* and *Canavalia* are mixed in equal proportion are boiled and made into a paste, which is soaked in a large container of water. The water is changed periodically for 15 days to remove the poisons. The water is changed until it removes the last trace of yellow colour. The mixture is dried and the white powder is eaten directly with flour or suguar or chilly powder. It cures several disorders and ensures good health.

Clitoria ternatea L.	*Sangu pushpam*	Paste of flowers applied to cure infection of eyes and for headache. Entire plant used as antidote for snake bites. Flowers offered to Gods.
Mucuna pruriens (L.) DC.	*Poonikali*	See '*Kozhiavarai* ' *Canavalia* lineata (Thunb.) DC.
Pongamia pinnata (L.) Pierre	*Pongan*	Seeds ground into paste and applied externally for knee and hip joints for rheumatic disease.
Tephrosia purpurea (L.) Pers.	*Averi*	Decoction of roots with ginger consumed to relieve headache.
Thespesia populnea (L.) Sol. ex Correa	*Poovarasu*	Yellow extract of fruit used for decorating houses.
Gentianaceae		
Enicostema axillare (Lam.) Raynal	*Vellarugu*	Secondary roots used as tooth brush to cure toothaches.
Lamaceae		
Geniosporum tenuiflorum (L.) Merr.*Leucas aspera* (Willd.) Link	*NilathulasiThumbai*	Paste of the plant mixed with limestone and applied to catfish bites.The thick roots are used as a tooth brush. Continuous use of a special preparation of this plant for 40 days makes one resistant to some snake poison. Flowers used during religious festivals.
Liliaceae		
Scilla hyacinthina (Roth.) Macbr. Contr.	*Narivangayam*	Bulbs used as substitute for onion.
Loranthaceae		
Dendrophthoe falcata (L.f.) Etting	*Ottai*	Fruits edible.

Marsileaceae		
Marsilea quadrifolia L.	*Aarakeerai*	Leaves used as green vegetable.
Meliaceae		
Azadirachta indica A. Juss.	*Veppam*	Tender leaf and bark extract consumed to eliminate stomach worms. Leaf twigs with leaves are tied or hanged in front of the house entrance to keep away evil spirits.
Minispermaceae		
Tiliacora acuminata (Lam.) Hook. f. & Thoms	*Perunkkattukodi*	Used as rope or binding bundles fuel woods.
Sapotaceae		
Mimusops elengi L.	Magizhamaram	Irulas name for this tree's flower is "Magishampoo". Irulas collect this flower from the forest and store them after they have been dried in the shade.
Tinospora cordifolia (Willd.) Miers	*Seenthil*	Stem and aerial roots ground into a fine powder and consumed with tea or nilk. It is used to cure many ailments.
Myrtaceae		
Syzygium cumini (L.) Skeels	*Naval*	Bark used for diarrhoea. The extract of bark mixed with goat milk and immediately consumed to stop diarrhoea.
Orchidaceae		
Cymbidium aloifolium (L.) Sw.	*Ottai*	Aerial root juice used as ear drop for relieving pain.

Pandanaceae		
Pandanus fascicularis Lam.	*Thazahi*	Silt roots used for making fibers and brushes. Fruits occasionally used as vegetable.
Poaceae		
Bambusa arundinacea (Retz.) Willd*Cynodon dactylon* (L.) Pers.	*MoongilArugampul*	Young shoots used as food. Stems used to build huts and spiritual ceremonies.Branches dipped in hot oil are used for a head-bath or as a body coolant.
Rhamnaceae		
Ziziphus mauritiana Lam.	*Elanthai*	Fruit edible. Powdered bark applied to old wounds.
Rubiaceae		
Catunaregam spinosa (Thunb.) Tirveng.	*Kattukoyya*	Fruit is cooked with other vegetables.
Rutaceae		
Toddalia asiatica (L.) Lam.	*Surai*	Decoction of leaves and stems used to controls fever. Fresh fruits eaten to reduce fever and headache.
Salvadoraceae		
Azima tetracantha Lam. *Salvadora persica* L.	*SankanVagai*	Leaves ground into pulp with water, the extract is used to treat a fever.Decoction of fruits and roots used to reduce rheumatic pains. Root used as tooth brush. Fruits commonly eaten.
Sapindaceae		
Cardiospermum halicacabum	*MudakkathanPoovanthi*	Whole plant used for treating rheumatoid

L.*Sapindus emarginatus* Vahl		arthritis.Wet ground nuts paste used for body wash as a surfactants
Sapotaceae		
Manilkara hexandra (Roxb.) Dubard	*Pala maram*	Latex applied on teeth and gums for toothaches. Fruits collected in large quantity and traded in local market for rice, chilli, tobacco, etc.
Scrophulariaceae		
Peplidium maritimum (L.f.) Asch.	*Parupu-keerai*	Leaves and tender stems consumed as food.
Simaroubaceae		
Ailanthus excelsa Roxb.	*Pekalathi*	A tonic prepared from the bark and leaves for healing after child birth.
Solanaceae		
Solanum anguivi Lam.	*Kandan kathiri*	Tender fruits cooked as vegetable and consumed for treating colds, coughs and fever. The tender leaves are made into a paste to treat intestinal worms.
Tamaricaceae		
Tamarix indica willd.	*Kattuchaukku*	Extract of leaves used as laxative.
Verbenaceae		
Gmelina asiatica L.	*Kumalai Nochi*	Fruits used as substitute for soap.Leaves repel
Vitex negundo L.		mosquitoes. Leaves boiled in water, which is used a bath to relieve body pain.

The most common plant families in the study were Euphorbiaceae (4 species) and Fabaceae (9 species) (complete list of families is given in Table below). Herbs (10 species) were the most common functional group of plants, followed by shrubs (13 species), climbers (10 species) and trees (17 species). A variety of plant morphological structures were utilized as medicine by the Irulas of which leaves were used most frequently, followed by roots, bark, seeds, whole plants, flowers, fruits and latex/sap. The preparation for utilization of these plant parts can be grouped into several categories based on the mode of preparation; decoction, extract, fresh or cooked plant, juice, latex, paste, and powder.

DIVERSITY IN IRULAS TK OF MEDICINAL PLANTS

The Irulas revealed ethnotaxa used to treat a variety of illnesses and promote general good health in their communities. TK of plants used to treat 30 illnesses were sorted into 12 usage categories, which were re-modified according to Cook and Heinrich. Plant remedies were utilized for various illness such as mosquito repellents, antibiotics, antidotes, appetizers, asthma, blood flow, body pain, body weak or feeble, cold, complementary food, cough, diabetes, diarrhoea, earache, eye pain, fever, general medicine, hydrocoele, hypothermia, intestinal worms, jaundice, leprosy, pregnancy pain, purgative, rheumatism, skin disease, skin-shine, spiritual, toothache and wounds. The diversity of ailments in our study may be limited to the common plants in our sample and some of the more common ailments treated in the Irulas villages, including ailments of mainstream people that come to the Irulas to be healed. Native healing practitioners provide a source of income for many Irulas families.

The Irulas shared the concept 'Neenda aauil', which translates to "living a long healthy life". The Irulas believe that the treatment of ailments can be pre-empted by a healthy life-style. The Irulas routinely consume plants for their vital well being and good health. Previous research indicates other cultures such as the Malasars that put a strong emphasis on daily consumption of plants to promote good health, which is supported by other studies that have recommended including the "general health" category in the standardized illness groupings. We included this category because it is an integral part of the Irulas health concept in which healers insist on having plants as part of their diet to maintain good health.

The general health category included the largest number of taxa, reports of utility and a relatively high level of consensus. We found in our survey that some of the plants used in the general health category are edible to the Irulas (8 species), while others were non-edible (19 species). The great variety of plants that are collected from the wild and distributed among the community or sent off to local markets for trading with other communities. An ancient tradition of the Irulas is to eat certain plants on a regular basis according to the seasons in order to prevent certain diseases. It is a common practice for the Irulas to consume plants in the wild throughout their daily routine. While hunting, the Irulas grab leaves of *Capparis zeylanica* L. and eat them fresh to stimulate their hunger and increase their desire to hunt. This plant is also served as an appetizer prepared as a dipping paste with pepper, tamarind and garlic. While trekking through the forest the Irulas would pick leaves to eat or chew on young tree branches; the forest is a natural pharmacopeia/grocery store for them.

The young Irulas are also engaged in the use of plants in their daily routine. Not unlike our modern society they encourage good hygiene at a young age. This may include cleaning or brushing your teeth with various types of young branches. However, we found that they combine both cleaning teeth at a young age with an ancient tradition called "priming". The Irulas believe that brushing your teeth with the roots of *thumbai* (*Leucas aspera* Willd.) for 40 consecutive days will make you immune to any snake venom. Called "priming", all children were once taught early in life to "prime" with *thumbai* before hunting snakes. Presently, very few elders in the Irulas community teach the practice of herbal immune priming to children.

One of the ailments that may be controlled by daily consumption of a particular plant is diabetes. Irulas have an ancient diagnostic system that utilizes their natural surroundings; to determine whether someone has *'Chakari noie'* (diabetes) the person is asked to urinate on the ground to see if ants are attracted to the abnormally high sugar concentration in their urine. The Irulas treat diabetes using an ethnotaxa called *'Sirukurinjan'*, which appears to be *Gymnema sylvestre* in the Asclepiadaceae or "milkweed family". The young, tender, shiny pale green leaves are preferred over the mature leaves, which will also be used. This TK was supported by high consensus among the informants (F_{ic} = 1.0).

Many Irulas families grow *Gymnema sylvestre* as a climbing vine near their home and it is a household custom to consume one leaf a day. They also regularly add leaves to several of the common curry dishes at least once a week even though the leaves add a bitter taste to the meal. If a young member if the household is diagnosed with *'Chakari noie'* (diabetes), they will be asked to consume 2 to 3 fresh tender leaves every morning before meals with a glass of water for about a year. Other research studies have documented *Gymnema sylvestre* as a natural remedy for diabetes. We recently recorded that the Malasars use *Gymnema sylvestre* for treating scorpion and rat bites, but do not use it to treat diabetes. Perhaps this is due to the fact that *Gymnema sylvestre* is not common at higher altitudes where the Malasars live.

The Irulas treat *'Moottu vadham'* (rheumatoid arthritis) with at least two different ethnotaxa, including *'Vagai'* and *'Mudakkathan'* both of which have a high consensus factor for the Irulas (F_{ic} = 1.0) within this study and by Malasars (F_{ic} = 0.78). The Malasars treat rheumatic pain using two other plants, *Diplocyclos palmatus* (L.) C. Jeffrey and *Boerhavia diffusa* L. We identified *'Mudakkathan'* to be *Cardiospermum halicacabum* L. *sensu lato* ('balloon vine') and *'Vagai'* to be *Salvadora persica* L. Previous research by Ragupathy revealed a complex taxonomy of several ethnotaxa for 'balloon vine', which has many associated utilities, including a remedy for joint pain. In many cultures this plant is harvested in backyards for both medicinal and food value. In fact, it provides an income supplement for some families from impoverished communities of third world countries.

The paradox is that *Cardiospermum halicacabum* is a poisonous (contains cyanide) invasive plant that agricultural researchers have described as a noxious weed that must be globally eradicated. We are currently investigating genetic variation among the haplotypes of *Cardiospermum halicacabum* and the complex cryptic taxonomy, which consists of several ethnotaxa.

Some modalities are less specific and are treated with a general all purpose plant such as '*Veeraii*', which means 'vigorous blood'. '*Veeraii*' has reddish sap and is used to treat '*Ratha o'ttam*' (blood circulation problems). We identified this ethnotaxa as *Diospyros ferrea* var. *buxifolia* (Wild.) Bahk. Previous research indicates that Malasars used '*Ratha surai*' (*Begonia malabarica* Roxb.), which also has reddish sap, to treat blood disorders. We had one record of the Irulas (an isolated mountain community near the Malasars), which used *Begonia malabarica Roxb.* to treat blood cancer. We assume that there are potential possibilities of knowledge sharing and further research is exploring variance in TK with respect different cultures and spatial scales.

The Irulas are also strong believers in spiritualism for which they utilize many plants. Although we will not report in detail plants used for spiritual reasons it is important to note that there was high consensus ($F_{ic} = 0.91$) among the informants for this utility category. We will briefly describe one application. We noticed that above every household doorway are a bunch of twigs tied in a bundle. This is '*Veppam*' (*Azadirachta indica* A. Juss.) and it is used to keep away evil sprits. Similarly, the Malasars who live in the mountain forest use plants ($F_{ic} = 0.87$), such as *Abrus precatorius* L., *Crotalaria verrucosa* and *Selaginella rupestris*, to repel-evil. There are several ethnotaxa used to repel evil and the preference for a particular ethnotaxa may be related to availability of the plant, but more likely the specific circumstances of the spiritual practice. Most treatments for folk illnesses can be found within cultural references; the Irulas treatment involves praying, communication with the evil sprit and the use of plants.

CONCLUSION

Throughout history aboriginal people have been the custodians of biodiversity while sustaining healthy life-styles that utilize natural resources. Unfortunately, their basic requirements sometimes force them into activities such as deforestation for monetary gains, or for extending agricultural activities that lead to a loss of biodiversity, which is the very source of their food and medicines. The Irulas are an excellent example of a culture that has not exploited a highly diverse area (KRF) despite the fact that they harvest their food and medicine from the wild for thousands of years. We have identified the reliable TK concerning the extent of the medicinal utility of plants by the Irulas that can be valorized using a consensus approach. This is the first step toward the recognition of TK in a scientific approach that will enhance society, nutrition, medicine, and resource management, etc.

A quantitative approach provides a means of validation and a measure of confidence. Clear methodology allows the research to be repeated and results to be applied at a larger scale to heal common ailments in society-at-large and use TK to understand biodiversity so that we can develop better management strategies and policies. We are currently conducting a study of the Irulas Traditional Ecological Knowledge (TEK) in order to understand their approach to ecosystem classification, conservation and sustainable utilization of natural resources.

The asymmetry between scientific and TK demands a new approach. We have identified the fact that ethnotaxa are not always synonymous with Linnaean taxonomy. In fact, TK has been used to expose cryptic diversity and discover new species that have utility to local cultures and must be considered within broader ecosystem management plans. However, these ethno-classification systems are very complicated and require a great deal of time to fully comprehend, reconstruct and utilize. This is a major impediment to engaging ethno-classification and the associated wealth of TK within the design of a comprehensive biodiversity study.

Modern automated identification technology (AIT), such as DNA barcoding, may provide a quick, repeatable and reliable tool for identifying ethnotaxa and variation in cryptic species. DNA barcoding is a method of species identification and recognition using specific regions of DNA sequence data. Recent development of an AIT system for plants indicates that the efficacy of an AIT system equates with savings in time and resources, while providing quick, reliable identifications. We are currently using DNA barcoding to discriminate the cryptic ethno-taxa for nutmegs, Acacia, Tripogon and within regional floras. We propose that a DNA barcode may be a quick and reliable tool to identify ethnotaxa, which will further legitimize the validity of TK, rendering it testable and ultimately generalisable, mobile and globally meaningful

One of our goals in this research is to document some of the Irulas TK using a science-based consensus approach. We were also able to protect this knowledge within our aboriginal repository of knowledge (ARK) research program and hope to develop educational programs within the Irulas communities. A greater understanding of TK is beginning to emerge based on our research with both the Irulas and Malasars; they believe that a healthy lifestyle is founded on a healthy environment. They chose to share this knowledge with society-at-large in order to promote a global lifestyle of health and environmental sustainability.

9

Crop Changes in Mountain Area of Eastern Liguria (Italy)

BACKGROUND

One frequent problem in assessing the causes and degree of changes in land use and crop diversity through time has been the scarcity of historical data for documenting such changes. Unfortunately, archival documentation has either not been preserved or is difficult to find, especially pertaining to periods prior to the XIX century.

The Council of Trent (1545–1563), introduced the bishops' requirement for periodic inspection of the inventories in each parish, convent or other ecclesiastic institution (including cultivated fields, forests, mills, etc.), encouraging their compilation. Such documents, used rarely in ethnobotanical investigation up to now, can be a very important source of chronological information on the composition and/or structure of agrocenoses and detailed features of land cover when specific for certain areas or even toponyms. Therefore, examination of the ecclesiastic possession inventories can enhance the knowledge of agricultural and livestock practice and subsistence methods of local populations during this time. In addition, other historical sources, such as cadastral maps, tax registers and manorial accounts, can give useful information about agricultural practices. Furthermore, indirect data regarding the natural environment (i.e. land cover) can be extrapolated from ancient archival documents.

It is well known that in past centuries subsistence agriculture was the main source of food for European people. Everywhere, cereals were the most important crop. Locally, cereals were partially replaced by other farm products, such as potatoes, legumes, olives, and chestnuts.

During the second half of the XX century, in many hill/ mountain regions of Europe (especially those close to the Mediterranean Sea) abandonment of mall-scale or household agriculture increased.

This abandonment occurred as humans began to systematically use extensive farming techniques, mostly in planned areas, and under the impacts of industrial/economic development.

Time-series investigations of changes in crop variety, even on a small scale, might uncover insights with broader regional implications.

In this chapter, we attempt to reconstruct changes in the type of crops and the characteristics of soil cover during the time from the XVI century to the present through archival and field research conducted on the inventories of the Parish of St. Mary and the Pignone territory in eastern Liguria.

METHODS

Study Area

The Municipality of Pignone lies in eastern Liguria, in Val di Vara, at the border with the National Park of the Cinque Terre, less than 10 kilometres from the Ligurian Sea; it rises 189 m above sea level.

The highest peak in the area reaches about 600 meters. In the study area, a Site of Community Importance (SCI), related to a karstic zone, is present.

From a historical point of view, the origin of Pignone village is very ancient, as indicated by archaeological findings from the Bronze Age on Mount Castellaro. The same name, "Castellaro", indicates the presence of Ligurian population settlements. In the Middle Ages, this area was the domain of the Malaspina dynasty, the bishops of Luni, the Fieschi dynasty and the Genova Republic.

The climate of the study area is sub-Mediterranean and characterised by warm summers and temperate winters; precipitation is mostly concentrated in spring and autumn.

From a phytogeographic point of view, the study area is located in the Italo-Thyrrenian province, within the Mediterranean region.

The natural vegetation present in the Pignone territory mainly consists of holm-oak (*Quercus ilex* L.) mixed woodland with a high cover of downy-oak (*Quercus pubescens* Willd.).

In a wide portion of the territory, cluster-pine (*Pinus pinaster* Aiton) anthropogenic and semi-natural (favoured by fire) woodlands are present.

On fresh slopes, a mixed woodland dominated by European hop-hornbeam (*Ostrya carpinifolia* Scop.), manna-ash (*Fraxinus ornus* L.) and downy-oak is present.

Locally, the vegetation is characterised by anthropogenic woods of chestnut (*Castanea sativa* Mill.). Black-alder (*Alnus glutinosa* (L.) Gaertn.) woodlands grow at the bottom of valleys, along with willow (*Salix* spp.) formations.

ARCHIVAL DATA AND FIELD SURVEY

In this study, five time periods since the XVI century are compared according to their crop or land use in the Pignone territory in the following years: 1588, 1663, 1763, 1828, 1878, 1933, and 2008.

The types of crops have been obtained through documentary investigation of all archival folders existing relating to the Parish of St. Mary in Pignone and to the Municipality of Pignone.

The former are stored in the "Niccolo V" Lunense Episcopal Archive of Sarzana (SP): series "Filze Parrocchiali". The latter are stored in the State Archive of La Spezia.

Table 1. Inventories (part A)

Inventories (part A)

Type of crop

Toponym	1588	1663	1763	1828	1878	1933	2008
A piè di Cravadora	Cg	Cg	Cg	Cg, W	x	x	Cg, W
Alla Focina	M	x	x	x	x	x	W
Alla Presa	x	Hf	x	x	x	Cg	x
Aretta	M	Hf	M, Ar	Al, Vy, Ar	x	x	W
Borela	x	x	x	Cg	x	W	B, W
Calcinarla 1	M	Hf	x	Al, Vy, Ar	Al, Vy, Ar	x	B
Calcinarla 2	M, Hf	Hf	M, Ar	Al, Vy, Ar	Al, Vy	Al, Vy	B, Al
*Campedio**	M	Og	x	x	x	x	x
Campuscasco 1	x	Cg	x	x	Cg, W	Cg, W	W
*Canavaro**	x	Hf	Hf	Al, Vy, Ar	x	Vy, Al	x
Carpena	Cg	x	x	x	x	x	x
*Coloreda 1**	Cg	Cg	Cg	Cg, W	x	W	Cg, W
Corasca	x	Cg	x	x	x	x	x
Coroni	Cg	x	x	x	x	x	x
Cravadora grande 1	Cg	Cg	Cg	Cg, W	Cg	W	W
Cravadora grande 2	Cg	Og	x	Cg, W	Cg, W	Cg, W	W
Cravadora minore 1	Cg	Cg	Cg	x	Cg	Cg, W	W
Cusanasco	x	Og	x	Al, Vy, Ar	x	x	x
Favà 1	Cg	Cg	Cg	Cg	Cg	Cg	Cg, W
*Fosicchia 1**	Cg, F	x	x	Cg, W	Cg	x	x
Il Castellaro 1	M	Og	Og	Og	Og, Cg	x	W
Il Castellaro di Bado	x	x	x	Og, Cg	x	x	W
Il Piaggio 1	x	Og	M, Ar	Cg, Al, W	M	M	W
Il Piaggio 2	x	Og	Og, Cg	Og, Cg	Og, Al	Al	W
Il Piaggio 3	x	x	x	Og, Cg, W	Cg	Al, Vy	W
Illegible toponym	M	x	x	x	x	x	x
Illegible toponym	x	Cg	x	x	x	x	x
Illegible toponym	x	x	Al, Ar	x	x	x	x
Illegible toponym	x	x	Cg	x	x	x	x
La Chiappara	Cg	x	Cg	x	Cg	x	x
La Chiosa 1	M, Vy, Ar	Vy	Cg, Ar, Vy, Al	Cg, Ar, Vy, Al	x	x	B, Al
La Chiosa 2	x	x	x	Cg	x	x	W
La dal Canale	x	x	x	Cg, W	Cg	Al, Vy	x
La Fornace	x	x	x	Al, Vy, Ar	x	x	x

La Giara	Hf*	Vy*	x	Al, Vy, Ar	x	Al	x
La Ligia	x	x	x	Cg, W	x	W, Cg	W
La Prata	x	x	x	Al, Vy, Ar	Al	x	x
La Ripalta	Cg	x	x	Cg, W	x	x	x
La Riva	x	x	x	Al, Vy, Ar	Al, Vy	x	x
Linà	x	Hf	Al, Ar	Cg	x	W	x
Linà	x	Og	x	x	x	x	x
*Madonna del Ponte 1**	x	Cg	Cg	Cg, W	x	W	W
Maggioli	x	x	x	Al, Vy, Ar	x	x	x
Nel Piano	M	x	x	x	Cg, M	x	x
Nel Trezzo	M	x	x	x	x	x	x
Patina	x	x	x	Cg	x	x	x
Pezza del Brazo	x	x	x	Al, Vy, Ar	x	x	x
Pezza del Molino	x	x	x	Al, Vy, Ar	x	Al	W
*Pezzo Grande 1**	M, Vy, Ar	x	x	Al, Vy, Ar	Vy, M, Ar, Al	x	x
Pian de Fossa 1	Cg	Cg	Cg	Cg, W	Cg	Cg	W
Piè di Favà	M	x	M, Ar	x	x	x	W
Piè di Favà	M*	x	M, Ar	x	x	x	W
Pignon soprano 1	M, Vy, Ar	Hf	Cg, Ar, Vy, Al	Cg, Ar, Vy, Al	x	Al, Vy, Cg	x
Pignon soprano 2	x	x	Cg, Ar, Vy, Al	x	x	Al, Vy, Cg	x
Pignon soprano 3	x	x	Cg, Ar, Vy, Al	x	x	x	x
Pignon soprano 4	x	x	Cg, Ar, Vy, Al	x	x	x	x
Pignon soprano 5	x	x	Cg, Ar, Vy, Al	x	Al	x	x
Pignon soprano 6	x	x	M	x	M	x	x
Pignon soprano 7	x	x	Og, Cg	x	x	x	x
Pilora 1	x	x	x	Al, Vy, Ar	x	Og	Og
Postemi	x	Cg	x	x	x	x	x
Rezzo 1	Cg	x	Ar	x	x	x	x
Rezzo 2	G	x	x	x	x	x	x
Rezzo 3	G*	Vy*	x	x	x	x	x
Rezzo 4	M	x	Ar	x	x	x	x
Rezzo 5	M	x	Ar	x	x	x	x
S. Antonio 1	x	x	x	Al, Vy, Ar	x	Og	W, Og
S. Michele	x	x	M, Ar	Al, Vy, Ar	x	x	x
*Scandolara 1**	Cg	Cg	Cg	x	x	Cg	W
Sotto la Lama	x	x	x	Al, Vy, Ar	x	x	x
Spinzo 1	x	Og	x	x	x	x	x
Spinzo 2	x	Og	x	x	x	x	x
Spinzo 3	x	Og	x	x	x	x	x
Sprugola A	Cg	x	Cg, M	x	x	x	x

Sprugola B	Cg	x	Cg	x	x	x	x
Su dal Canale	x	x	x	Cg, W	x	x	x
Tra la Chiesa	M	x	Og, Cg	x	x	x	W, Vy
Tra le case	M	Hf	M	x	x	x	x
Va' 1	x	x	x	Cg	Cg	Cg	x
Vaccheredo	Cg	x	x	x	x	x	x

Inventories, ordered for every toponym, of the Parish of St. Mary and of the Municipality of Pignone, for the years 1588, 1663, 1763, 1828, 1878, 1933 and recent times. Part A comprises toponyms listed in the ecclesiastic inventories (years 1588, 1663, 1763, 1828). Legend: Ar = arboretum; B = buildings; Cg = chestnut grove; Hf = hempfield; G = grassland; M = meadow; Og = olive grove; Al = arable land; W = woodland; Vy = vineyard; * = include a mill; x: no data.

Table 2. Inventories (part B)

Inventories (part B)

Type of crop

Toponym	1588	1663	1763	1828	1878	1933	2008
Ai Laghi 1	x	x	x	x	W	Al	Al
Ai Laghi 2	x	x	x	x	x	Al, Vy	Al, Vy
Alle Noci	x	x	x	x	x	W	W
Bandita	x	x	x	x	x	W	W
Banzola 1	x	x	x	x	Cg	W, Cg	W
Banzola 2	x	x	x	x	W	W	W
Banzola 3	x	x	x	x	W	W	W
Banzola 4	x	x	x	x	x	W	W
Battipagliano 1	x	x	x	x	Cg	Cg	Cg
Battipagliano 2	x	x	x	x	Al	Al	x
Battipagliano 3	x	x	x	x	Al, Cg	Cg, M	Cg, W
Battipagliano 4	x	x	x	x	Vy, Al	Al	W
Battipagliano 5	x	x	x	x	Vy, Al	Al	W
Battipagliano 6	x	x	x	x	x	Al	Al
Battipagliano 7	x	x	x	x	x	Al, M	Al, M
Bogiolo	x	x	x	x	x	Al	Al

Borale 1	x	x	x	x	Vy, Al	Al	Al
Borale 2	x	x	x	x	Vy, Al, Og	x	W
Borale 3	x	x	x	x	Vy, Al	x	W
Borale 4	x	x	x	x	Al, Vy	x	M
Borale 5	x	x	x	x	Cg	x	B, W
Bosco del Gallino	x	x	x	x	W	x	W
Calcinarla 3	x	x	x	x	W	x	B, Al
Calcinarla 4	x	x	x	x	Al, Vy, irrig	Al	B, Al
Calcinarla 5	x	x	x	x	Cg	x	B, Al
Calcinarla 6	x	x	x	x	Al, Vy	Al, Vy, Cg	B, Al
Calcinarla 7	x	x	x	x	Al, Vy	Al	B, Al
Calcinarla 8	x	x	x	x	Al, Vy	x	B, Al
Calcinarla 9	x	x	x	x	Al, Vy	x	B, Al
Campuscasco 2	x	x	x	x	Cg	x	W
Cantarana	x	x	x	x	Al, Vy	x	x
Castellino	x	x	x	x	x	W	x
Cerreta	x	x	x	x	x	Cg, W	x
Cerreta	x	x	x	x	Og	W	x
Ciazzo	x	x	x	x	Vy, Al	x	x
Colorede 2	x	x	x	x	W	W	Cg, W
Costa dell'Olivella	x	x	x	x	Cg	x	W
Cravadora 1	x	x	x	x	Cg	Cg, W	W
Cravadora 2	x	x	x	x	W	W	W
Cravadora 3	x	x	x	x	Cg	Cg	W
Cravadora 4	x	x	x	x	Cg	W	W
Cravadora 5	x	x	x	x	Cg	W	W
Cravadora 6	x	x	x	x	Cg	W	W
Cravadora 7	x	x	x	x	Cg	Cg, W	W
Cravadora di Sotto	x	x	x	x	W, Cg	W	W, Cg
Cravadora minore 2	x	x	x	x	Cg	W	W
Cuccaro 1	x	x	x	x	Al, Vy, Ar	W	W
Cuccaro 10	x	x	x	x	Cg	Cg	Cg
Cuccaro 2	x	x	x	x	Al	W	W
Cuccaro 3	x	x	x	x	Cg	W	W, Cg
Cuccaro 4	x	x	x	x	Al, Vy, Ar	Al, Vy, Cg	Al

Cuccaro 5	x	x	x	x	Al	Al, Vy	Vy
Cuccaro 6	x	x	x	x	Al	W	W
Cuccaro 7	x	x	x	x	Cg	Cg, W	W
Cuccaro 8	x	x	x	x	Al, Vy	Al, Vy	Al, Vy
Cuccaro 9	x	x	x	x	Al	W	W
Cuneo 1	x	x	x	x	x	Al, W	Al, W
Cuneo 2	x	x	x	x	x	W	x
Cuneo sottano 1	x	x	x	x	x	Al	x
Cuneo sottano 2	x	x	x	x	x	W, Al	x
Cusidore	x	x	x	x	W	x	W
Due Canali 1	x	x	x	x	x	Cg	x
Due Canali 2	x	x	x	x	x	Cg	x
Due Canali 3	x	x	x	x	x	Cg	x
Favà 2	x	x	x	x	Cg, Og	Cg	Cg, W
Favà 3	x	x	x	x	Cg, Og	W	W
Filagne	x	x	x	x	Al	x	x
Fontanella 1	x	x	x	x	Cg, W	x	Cg, W
Fontanella 2	x	x	x	x	Cg, W	x	Cg, W
Fontanella 3	x	x	x	x	W	x	W
*Fosicchia 2**	x	x	x	x	Cg	Cg	x
*Fosicchia 3**	x	x	x	x	Cg	Cg	x
Fossalonga	x	x	x	x	Cg	x	x
Foxina 1	x	x	x	x	M	Al	x
Foxina 2	x	x	x	x	Al, Vy	Al	x
Foxina 3	x	x	x	x	x	Al	x
Foxina 4	x	x	x	x	x	Al	x
Foxina Grande	x	x	x	x	x	Al, Vy	x
Frantoio 1	x	x	x	x	x	Al, Vy	x
Frantoio 2	x	x	x	x	x	Al, Vy	x
Frantoio 3	x	x	x	x	x	Al	x
Frantoio 4	x	x	x	x	x	Al	x
Frassaneda	x	x	x	x	x	W	x
Gaggiolo	x	x	x	x	Cg, Al	W	x
Garzarelli	x	x	x	x	x	W	x
Grizzola 1	x	x	x	x	Vy, Ar, Al	W, Cg	W, Cg

Grizzola 2	x	x	x	x	Cg, Og	Al, Vy, Og, Cg	W, Cg
Grizzola 3	x	x	x	x	Al	Cg	W, Cg
Grizzola 4	x	x	x	x	Cg	Cg	W, Cg
Grizzola 5	x	x	x	x	Cg	Cg	W, Cg
Grizzola 6	x	x	x	x	Cg, Og, Al	Cg	W
Grizzola 7	x	x	x	x	x	Al, Vy, Og	Al, Vy, Og
Il Campo 1	x	x	x	x	Vy, Ar, Al	Al	x
Il Campo 2	x	x	x	x	Vy, Ar, Al	Al, Vy	x
Il Campo 3	x	x	x	x	Al	Al	x
Il Campo 4	x	x	x	x	Vy, Al, Cg	Cg	x
Il Castellaro 2	x	x	x	x	Og	x	W
Il Giardino	x	x	x	x	Al, Vy	x	x
Il Piaggio 4	x	x	x	x	Al	Al	x
Il Piaggio 5	x	x	x	x	x	Al	x
Il Piaggio 6	x	x	x	x	x	Og, Al	x
Lama di Pianello	x	x	x	x	Cg, W	x	x
*Madonna del Ponte 2**	x	x	x	x	Cg	Cg	W
*Madonna del Ponte 3**	x	x	x	x	Cg	x	W, Cg
Migiaro	x	x	x	x	Cg	x	W, Cg
Migliarese 1	x	x	x	x	Cg	Cg	W, Cg
Migliarese 2	x	x	x	x	Cg	Cg	W, Cg
Migliarese 3	x	x	x	x	x	W	W
Migliarese 4	x	x	x	x	x	Cg	W
Migliarese 5	x	x	x	x	x	Cg	W
Migliarese 6	x	x	x	x	x	W	W
Migliarese 7	x	x	x	x	x	W	W
Migliarese 8	x	x	x	x	x	W	W
Migliarese di sopra	x	x	x	x	x	W	W
Migliarese di sotto	x	x	x	x	x	Cg, W	W
Monteletto 1	x	x	x	x	Og, Vy, Al	M	x
Monteletto 2	x	x	x	x	Og, Vy, Al	x	x
Monteletto 3	x	x	x	x	Vy, Og, Cg	x	x
Monteletto 4	x	x	x	x	Cg	x	x
Mostani	x	x	x	x	Cg, W	x	x
Narneia Grande 1	x	x	x	x	x	W	x

Narneia Grande 2	x	x	x	x	x	W	x
Olivella	x	x	x	x	Cg	x	W
Orto 1	x	x	x	x	x	Al	x
Orto 2	x	x	x	x	x	Al, Vy	x
Orto 3	x	x	x	x	x	Al, Vy	x
Pastine 1	x	x	x	x	Al, Vy	Al, Vy	Al, Vy
Pastine 2	x	x	x	x	Cg	Vy, Cg	Cg
Pastine 3	x	x	x	x	Cg	Vy, Al	Vy, Al
Pastine 4	x	x	x	x	Cg, W	x	Cg, W
Pastine 5	x	x	x	x	Vy, Ar, Al	x	Cg, W
Pastine 6	x	x	x	x	x	Al, Vy, Cg	Cg, W
Perlo 1	x	x	x	x	Og, Cg	Og, Cg	W
Perlo 2	x	x	x	x	x	Al	W, Cg
Perlo 3	x	x	x	x	x	W, Cg	W, Cg
Perlo 4	x	x	x	x	x	Al, Cg	W
Perlo 5	x	x	x	x	x	Og	W
Perlo 6	x	x	x	x	x	Al, Og, Cg	W
*Pezzo Grande 2**	x	x	x	x	Vy, Al	x	x
Pian de Fossa 10	x	x	x	x	x	Cg	W
Pian de Fossa 2	x	x	x	x	x	Cg	W, Cg
Pian de Fossa 3	x	x	x	x	Al	Cg	W, Cg
Pian de Fossa 4	x	x	x	x	Al, Cg	Al, Vy, Cg	W
Pian de Fossa 5	x	x	x	x	Cg	Cg	W
Pian de Fossa 6	x	x	x	x	Cg	Cg	W
Pian de Fossa 7	x	x	x	x	Cg	Cg	W
Pian de Fossa 8	x	x	x	x	Cg	Cg	W
Pian de Fossa 9	x	x	x	x	x	Og	W
Pian di Casa	x	x	x	x	x	Al	x
Pian di Manin	x	x	x	x	x	Al, M	x
Piana di Gatella	x	x	x	x	Cg	x	x
Piano del Ponte rotto	x	x	x	x	x	Al	x
Piazzale	x	x	x	x	Vy, Al, Cg	Vy, Al	x
Pignon sottano 1	x	x	x	x	Al	Al	x
Pignon sottano 2	x	x	x	x	Vy, Ar, Al	x	x
Pignon sottano 3	x	x	x	x	Al, Vy	Al, Vy	x

Pignon sottano 4	x	x	x	x	Vy, Ar, Al	x	x
Pignon sottano 5	x	x	x	x	Vy, Al	Vy, Al	x
Pignon sottano 6	x	x	x	x	Vy, Al	Vy, Al	x
Pignon sottano 7	x	x	x	x	Vy, Al	Vy, Al	x
Pignon sottano 8	x	x	x	x	Vy, Al	x	x
Pilora 2	x	x	x	x	x	Og	W
Pilora 3	x	x	x	x	x	Og	W
Pilora 4	x	x	x	x	x	Al	W
Porcile	x	x	x	x	Vy, M, Ar, Al	x	x
Porcinasco	x	x	x	x	Al	x	x
Possessione 1	x	x	x	x	Al	Al, Vy, Cg	Al, Vy, Cg
Possessione 2	x	x	x	x	x	Al, Vy	Al, Vy
Possessione 3	x	x	x	x	x	Al, Vy	Al, Vy
Pradiera 1	x	x	x	x	Ar, Vy, Al	x	x
Pradiera 2	x	x	x	x	Vy, Al	x	x
Pradiera 3	x	x	x	x	Al	Al	x
Pradiera 4	x	x	x	x	Al	Al	x
Pradiera 5	x	x	x	x	Al	x	x
Pradiera 6	x	x	x	x	Al	x	x
Prati Grandi 1	x	x	x	x	x	Al	x
Prati Grandi 2	x	x	x	x	x	Al	x
Prati Grandi 3	x	x	x	x	x	Al	x
Prato Longo 1	x	x	x	x	Al, Cg	Al	x
Prato Longo 2	x	x	x	x	Al	Al	x
Prato Longo 3	x	x	x	x	x	Al	x
Rivone 1	x	x	x	x	Cg, Al, Vy	Cg, Al, Vy	x
Rivone 2	x	x	x	x	x	Al	x
Rivone 3	x	x	x	x	x	Al, Vy	x
S. Antonio 2	x	x	x	x	x	Og	W
S. Antonio 3	x	x	x	x	x	Og	W
Saggiano 1	x	x	x	x	Cg	x	W
Saggiano 2	x	x	x	x	Al, Cg	x	W
Saggiano 3	x	x	x	x	W	x	W
Saggiano 4	x	x	x	x	Cg, W, Al	x	W
Saramazzo 1	x	x	x	x	Al, Vy	Al, Vy	Al, Vy

Saramazzo 2	x	x	x	x	Al, Og	Al	Al
Saramazzo 3	x	x	x	x	Al, Vy	Al, Vy	Al, Vy
Saramazzo 4	x	x	x	x	Al, Vy	Al, Vy	Al, Vy
Saramazzo 5	x	x	x	x	Al, Vy	Al	Al
Saramazzo 6	x	x	x	x	x	Al	Al
Saramazzo 7	x	x	x	x	x	Al, Vy, Cg	W
Saramazzo 8	x	x	x	x	x	Al, Vy	Al, Vy
Saramazzo 9	x	x	x	x	x	Al, Vy	Al, Vy
*Scandolara 2**	x	x	x	x	x	Cg, W	W
*Scandolara 3**	x	x	x	x	x	W	W
*Scandolara 4**	x	x	x	x	x	W, Cg	W
*Scandolara 5**	x	x	x	x	x	W	W
Scoglio del Zer	x	x	x	x	Ar (walnut)	x	x
Selva	x	x	x	x	W	x	x
Serralunga	x	x	x	x	x	W	x
Suasca	x	x	x	x	x	Cg, W	x
Taramasco 1	x	x	x	x	Cg	x	x
Taramasco 2	x	x	x	x	Al	x	x
Termini	x	x	x	x	Al	x	W
Tra la Serra	x	x	x	x	Al, Vy	Al, Vy	x
Tra le coste 1	x	x	x	x	Vy, Ar, Al	W	x
Tra le coste 10	x	x	x	x	x	Al, Cg	x
Tra le coste 11	x	x	x	x	x	Cg, Al	x
Tra le coste 2	x	x	x	x	Al	Al	x
Tra le coste 3	x	x	x	x	Vy, Ar, Al	Al	x
Tra le coste 4	x	x	x	x	Al	Al	x
Tra le coste 5	x	x	x	x	Cg, Vy	Cg	x
Tra le coste 6	x	x	x	x	Cg, W	Cg	x
Tra le coste 7	x	x	x	x	Cg	Cg	x
Tra le coste 8	x	x	x	x	Vy, M, Al	Vy, Cg	x
Tra le coste 9	x	x	x	x	x	Al	x
Tra le coste di sopra	x	x	x	x	x	Cg	x
Tra le coste di sotto	x	x	x	x	x	Al, Cg	x
Tra le vigne	x	x	x	x	x	Cg, W	x
Trombassa	x	x	x	x	x	Cg, W	x
Va' 2	x	x	x	x	Cg, Og	Cg, Og	x

Va' 3	x	x	x	x	Cg	Cg, W	x
Va' 4	x	x	x	x	Og	Og	x
Va' 5	x	x	x	x	Al	W	x
Va' 6	x	x	x	x	Cg, Og	W	x
Va' 7	x	x	x	x	Vy, W	W	x
Va' 8	x	x	x	x	Al, Og	Og	x
Va' 9	x	x	x	x	Og	Og	x
Va' 10	x	x	x	x	Vy, Ar, Al	x	x
Va' 11	x	x	x	x	Al, Og	Al, Og	x
Val del Gallo 1	x	x	x	x	Vy, Ar, Al	x	x
Val del Gallo 2	x	x	x	x	Vy, Ar, Al	x	x
Val del Gallo 3	x	x	x	x	Vy, Ar, Al	x	x
Val del Gallo 4	x	x	x	x	Al	x	x
Val del Rio	x	x	x	x	Al, W	x	x
Val di Franeta 1	x	x	x	x	W	W	W
Val di Franeta 2	x	x	x	x	x	W	W
Val di Becco 1	x	x	x	x	Cg, W	x	x
Val di Becco 2	x	x	x	x	W	x	x
Valdelloro 1	x	x	x	x	Cg	x	W, Cg
Valdelloro 2	x	x	x	x	W	W	W
Valdelloro 3	x	x	x	x	W	W	W
Valdelloro 4	x	x	x	x	W	x	W
Valdelloro 5	x	x	x	x	W, Cg	W, Cg	W
Valdelloro 6	x	x	x	x	W, Cg	W, Cg	W
Valdelloro 7	x	x	x	x	Cg, W	W	W
Valetti	x	x	x	x	x	W	W
Valle	x	x	x	x	x	Al	x
Valle della Vecchia	x	x	x	x	Cg	Cg, W	W
Valle di Vallone	x	x	x	x	x	Cg, W	x
Valle Grande 1	x	x	x	x	x	W	x
Valle Grande 2	x	x	x	x	x	W	x
Vanedi 1	x	x	x	x	Al, Vy	M	x
Vanedi 2	x	x	x	x	x	Al	x
Vanzola	x	x	x	x	x	W	x
Varcava 1	x	x	x	x	Cg	x	W
Varcava 2	x	x	x	x	W	x	W

Inventories, ordered for every toponym, of the Municipality of Pignone, for the years 1878, 1933 and recent times.

Analysis of aerial photographs and field surveys allowed the investigation of current land use (crops, natural vegetation, buildings).

Ancient toponyms listed in the inventories were compared with current ones that can be found in the cadastral map of the Municipality of Pignone. A complete correlation between ancient and current toponyms does not exist: the former, in part, have been lost; in some cases, more than one type of crop exists for a single toponym.

The antique inventories were written in ancient Italian. Hence the following words, which were found singly or together and linked to toponyms or individually, were annotated:

- Arboretum (Ar): field planted, probably with fruit trees, such as walnut (*Juglans regia* L.), fig (*Ficus carica* L.), apple (*Malus domestica* (Borkh.) Borkh.), etc.;
- Buildings (B): area occupied by recent buildings (houses, parking, ways, etc);
- Chestnut grove (Cg): anthropogenic woods of chestnut (*Castanea sativa*), frequently in terrace cultivation.
- Meadow (M): land, probably held for forage production;
- Grassland (G);
- Hempfield (Hf): farmland for hemp (*Cannabis sativa* L.);
- Olive grove (Og): land planted with olives (*Olea europaea* L.), often in terrace cultivation;
- Woodland (W): vegetation to forest (*Quercus* spp., *Pinus pinaster*, *Ostrya carpinifolia*, *Fraxinus ornus*, *Salix* spp., etc.);
- Arable land (Al): very probably crops with wheat (*Triticum* spp.), barley (*Hordeum vulgare* L.) and rye (*Secale cereale* L.); in more recent times, maize (*Zea mays* L.) or vegetables, such as broad bean (*Vicia faba* L.), pea (*Pisum sativum* L.) and chick pea (*Cirer arietinum* L.).
- Vineyard (Vy): land planted with vines (*Vitis vinifera* L.).

The percent frequency of all crop portions (type) were computed for each inventory.

The relationship between the total number of fields (referred to as toponyms) and the total number of crop portions (for all fields) have been calculated for each inventory as an indicator of crop uniformity (CU). The botanical nomenclature used in this paper follows.

Results

In the "Niccolo V" Lunense Episcopal Archive of Sarzana, four inventories related to the Parish of St. Mary in Pignone were found and transcribed. The first archival documents date back to 1588; the next date back to 1663, 1763 and 1828.

Year 1588

Fields for forage production (meadow) and chestnut grove prevail. Other crop types are scarce. The relationship between the number of fields (38) and the number of crop portions (CU: 38/46) is 0.83.

Year 1663

Chestnut groves prevail, with a small decrease in the total number of fields from 16 (in 1588) to 12. In the XVII century, olive cultivation, not mentioned in the previous inventory, seems to have become extensive. Hemp cultivation increases (from 1 to 8 fields). Three crops cultivated on the vine are present. The CU indicator is 1 (33/33), as all inventoried fields are utilized for only one crop type.

Year 1763

Chestnut groves prevail in this period as well. A fair number of fields with mixed cultures are present with chestnut groves, arboretums, vineyards and arable lands. There is a decrease in areas planted exclusively with olive crops. The CU indicator is 0.56 (36/64).

Year 1828

Mixed cultures with vine, arboretum and arable land prevailing. There was a substantial decrease in fields with exclusive chestnut production, but increased mixed areas with chestnut groves and woods. The CU indicator is 0.43 (41/95), the lowest value among the inventories studied. In the State Archive of La Spezia, two inventories related to the Municipality of Pignone were found and transcribed. The archival documents date back to 1878 and 1933.

Year 1878

Arable land seems to be the main kind of crop, along with chestnut groves with an increase with respect to the previous (ecclesiastic) inventory. Woodlands are almost stable. On the other hand, the relationship between the number of fields and the number of crop (CU) portions increased to 0.61 (194/316).

Year 1933

Arable land prevail. There was a substantial decrease in fields with chestnut groove and a increase of woods. The CU indicator is 0.73 (226/311).

Current

To monitor the present landscape and crops, field surveys were carried out with the help of aerial photographs and the cadastral map of the Pignone territory. This allowed us to compare present and past situations linked to specific toponyms. The majority of ancient fields with chestnut groves and olive groves have been abandoned and partially reforested with cluster-pine woodland or mixed coppiced woodland (oaks, chestnuts, European hop-hornbeam, etc.). Some areas now have buildings.

At the other sites in Pignone, not linked to the toponyms noted in the inventories, a general reforestation has been surveyed. Vineyards and olive groves at present have been on the whole abandoned. The few arable lands consist of maize or vegetables. The CU indicator is 0.75 (168/224).

Discussion

Ecclesiastic institutions were among the main landowners in Europe until the end of the XIX century. For this reason, such inventory data gives us qualitative and semiquantitative information regarding the types of crop change throughout time in an area of eastern Liguria. After the XIX century, data from the inventories of municipalities and from forest inventories are available for the same territory. Such information is in agreement with historical knowledge related to the study area and to other Mediterranean hill/mountain areas.

The chestnut, in historical times, was spread by Romans as plant for food. However, it is well documented that starting in the Middle Ages chestnut cultivation spread throughout the Mediterranean hill/mountain areas of Italy (then in Val di Vara), replacing part of the holm-oak woods. In Val di Vara, domestication of the woodland chestnut tree spread during the XIV century, along with a strong increase in population.

Our data confirm such assertions and show that the main subsistence means in the study area from the XVI century to the first half of the XIX century was chestnut, and secondarily meadow in 1588, hempfield and olive in 1663, arboretum in 1763 and vine in 1828. In the study area in 1878 and 1933, arable land prevailed along with chestnut groves. High values of the CU indicator have evidenced few diversified crops in the XVI and XVII centuries. Crop diversification increased until the first half of the XIX century (low values of the CU indicator), then it decreased again (high values of the CU indicator).

In addition, in other Mediterranean regions, chestnut has been a tree historically cultivated and utilized as food, but also for a variety of other practices. For example, chestnut could be utilized around crops in lines together with other trees as a barrier to wind, to stabilize soil and to support the harvest of leaves and branches for livestock. In vineyards, vines were generally sustained by chestnut poles arranged in rows or pergolas.

In the study area and during some periods, a lesser part was played by olives and vines in agricultural activities. On the contrary, in the warmer areas of the Mediterranean basin close to the coast, olive groves and vineyards were the main crop types.

General investigation of the Ligurian Republic dated back to 1799 and supplied data regarding forest vegetation and crop types in Val di Vara (some locations). For example, in the nearby Val di Pino, holm-oak and chestnut crops were present.

In other locations in Val di Vara (San Pietro Vara and Varese Ligure) fields of chestnut, turkey-oak (*Quercus cerris* L.), downy-oak, European hop-hornbeam, beech (*Fagus sylvatica* L.), willow trees (*Salix* spp.) and olive trees were noted. Crops with major production indices included chestnut, followed by wine, olive oil, wheat, rye, fruits, figs, legumes, potatoes (*Solanum tuberosum* L.), and vegetables. Particularly interesting is the earlier presence of cultivated potatoes in Val di Vara. In Italy, the potato was introduced in Genova around 1585 by Carmelite Friars from Spain and Portugal. However, the potato had begun to spread throughout all of Europe, and in eastern Liguria starting from the second half of the XVIII century. Around Genova to the Val di Vara territory, the variety "Quarantina bianca" was cultivated. The progressive increase in the cultivation and utilisation of potato and maize is considered one of the causes of the decrease in nutritional importance of the chestnut tree starting from the second half of the XIX century. Our data support this assertion, as in the inventories of 1878 and 1933 arable land (Al) were the main crop type.

Starting from the XIX century (inventory of 1828), there was an increase of woodlands. This was very probably due to a transformation in the socio-economic conditions and also to the production of coal inside charcoal pits. This practice disappeared everywhere after the Second World War, but gaps produced by the old charcoal spaces persist and are still visible in the woods. In eastern Liguria (also in the Pignone territory), there has been increased extractive activities in this century in several modest mines for industrial, energy or building purposes, such as pyrite, kaolin, lignite, and sandstone. Such activity locally favoured the exploitation of the woods in the areas close to the mines.

Since the first half of the XIX century, chestnut ink disease, caused by *Phytophthora cambivora* and *P. cinnamomi* has become widespread in Europe. In Italy and particularly in eastern Liguria, ink disease and chestnut disease (cancer of the bark) gravely damaged chestnut groves starting from the end of the XIX century until about 1950.

Before the XX century, the agricultural system in the study area mainly produced food for self-sustaining local communities, parishes and landowners, and only occasionally for external commerce.

During the XX century, chestnut groves in the study area significantly decreased in importance. Such trends have been evidenced in upper Val di Vara: in 1938, the chestnut woods (coppiced and trees) covered about 60% of the territory. After the Second World War, in Val di Vara there were strongly augmented plantations of the most degraded woodland (erosion) with coniferous trees. In 1993, most of the territory was forested by mixed woodlands, turkey-oak woodlands and plantations (*Pinus* spp.), and only 15% of the area was occupied by chestnut coppice.

The recent forest census of the Liguria Region revealed that only about 22% of the forest surface of the whole Province of La Spezia is occupied by chestnut (comprising coppice); mixed coppiced woodland and cluster pine woodland represent 21.8% and 15.2% respectively. The same forest census showed that in the Pignone territory, chestnut coppice represents 20%, mixed woodland 27.60% (oaks, chestnuts, European hop-hornbeam, etc.), cluster pine woodland 13.1%, olive grove 2.5%, and other cultivated lands 9.7%.

In this context, the traditional elements of the rural landscape, in terms of chestnut groves and olive groves (terraces, stonewalls, etc.), have been not preserved, but rather have deteriorated or been destroyed. We can assert that agriculture abandonment and changing socio-economic conditions over the last 50 years have favoured a strong increase in cluster-pine woodland or mixed coppiced woodland (oaks, chestnuts, European hop-hornbeam, etc.) and partially in evergreen sclerophyllous forest and shrubland at the expense of cultivated areas, especially those with chestnuts and olives. A similar trend has been observed for coastal areas of eastern Liguria, where vineyard, the dominant crop type, has been mainly substituted by cluster pine woodland.

As evidenced in other Mediterranean hill/mountain areas, this has lead to a simplification of the landscape (an increase in the CU indicator) due to abandonment of agricultural practices and reforestation.

Conclusion

This study has examined crop/land cover changes during the last five centuries in an area of eastern Liguria (Italy) through examination of archival documents taken from ecclesiastic and municipal inventories, and current field surveys. In accordance with other studies conducted in the Mediterranean region, we show evidence of the traditional use of chestnut as one of the main source of food in the hill/mountain areas of eastern Liguria in the XVI, XVII and XVIII centuries. This work has highlighted how ancient documents, which are at present not generally used in ethnobotanical studies, can be very useful for enhancing the knowledge of agricultural and livestock practices and of subsistence methods favoured by local populations during a particular time. This study has also shown that inventories (but also other types of documents) are very useful for the historical reconstruction of the landscape by means of relative comparison of cultivated fields, anthropogenic woods and naturally reforested areas.

10

Extending the Temporal Context of Ethnobotanical Databases

BACKGROUND

In the last decade, several information systems have been developed to collect and manage the traditional knowledge (TK) on the use of plants from different geographical areas. As far as the Mediterranean basin is concerned, networks like MEDUSA have been established to identify native and naturalized plants, and to set up an on-line database. In the same area the integrated and multi-disciplinar project RUBIA focuses on the collection and dissemination of TK related to uses of wild and neglected cultivated plants, also exploring the relationships to folkloric history and socio-cultural context.

On a wider geographical scale, Thomas et al. developed an electronic archive based on object database technology for submission, storage and retrieval of ethnomedicinal data, and Skoczen and Bussmann have recently presented their International Ethnobotany Database (ebDB), an on-line database, which provides a generic solution for ethnobotanical data storage, being multilingual, and open to anyone wants to add information. Although those databases implement advanced solutions regarding linguistic and semantic issues, they have not been designed for the storage of data ranging over large temporal extensions, and, at present, no data base repository has been specifically developed with a focus on historical ethnobotany.

It has been recently stressed that one of the unresolved problems of the present ethnobotanical and ethnopharmacological studies is the limited contribution of disciplines like anthropology and historical sciences. As a consequence the focus of ethnobotanical research is rarely given by the comprehension of the traditional health systems and their development during the centuries.

On the other hand, the complexity of this approach requires adequate tools to manage the complex flow of information collected. The historical complexity, common to Mediterranean area, requires an integrated approach to understand the context and the evolution of local traditional knowledge on plant uses. As a case-study, we selected the Campania region (southern Italy), which has been inhabited since prehistoric times by different ethnic groups, thus merging different traditions into a unique *corpus* of traditional knowledge. Before the Roman colonization, Greek and Etrurian colonies occupied this region, together with indigenous Italic people, as Osci and Samnites. Later on, the Region of Campania was annexed by the Romans and, after the fall of the Western Roman Empire, different populations ranging from Goths and Byzantines, to Arabs, Normans and Longobards occupied part of the territory or established lasting relationships with local populations.

A relational database has been elaborated with the goal of providing a standard for the storage of historical series of ethnobotanical data in the Mediterranean region, allowing the temporal exploration of links and meanings.

Methods

Development of the database

The database prototype has been implemented as a local relational database. Different implementation solutions were tested, according to the requirements and use cases. Present and ancient ethnobotanical data were organized in the same table structure, allowing some costs of redundancy in favor of the homogenization of data and queries. Because flexibility was a major issue for our archive, object oriented concepts were implemented, such as unlimited hierarchical structures (self-joined tables), particularly for categorized look-up tables and species taxonomy, and inheritance concepts, allowing e.g. information sources to be a reference, a person, an herbal or an archeological remain. Those techniques allowed us to develop a minimal data structure fitting different kind of information, and to perform queries at different levels of detail.

Table: Short description of the tables of the database

Table Name	Description
Ethnobotanical relevée	Details of the ethnobotanical relevée, like site, coordinates, source (e.g. collector) and spatial relevance. This relevée can then contain information on multiple plants.
Plant	Information relative to the plant, like reference to the phytonym, source (e.g. informant), reliability of the phytonym identification and general notes. A plant can then contain details on multiple uses.
Plant use	Information on the use of the plant, namely classified use and use category, use description and reliability (especially for information from the ancient treatises or archeological remains).
Plant preparation	The preparation of the plant is stored according to preparation mode and plant part used. Multiple steps for the preparation of a single plant use (receipt) can also be recorded.
Phytonym	Different phytonyms, of different types. In this table are stored also the scientific names, including synonyms.
Taxon assignment	Join table storing the taxon assignments to the phytonyms, with the source and the reliability. For the case of scientific phytonyms, and for most of the Italian phytonyms, the reliability is considered sure.A phytonym can have multiple putative identifications.
Taxon	Scientific name of the taxon, organized in a hierarchical structure (at different taxonomic levels), e.g. Labiatae > Thymus > Thymus serpyllum. Only

	the accepted scientific synonym is stored in this table.
Specimen	Herbal specimen information.
Herbal collection	Details on the herbal collection.
Life form	Different life forms, organized in a hierarchical structure (with different detail levels), e.g. Therophytes > erect.
Phytonym type	Ancient, Italian, popular and scientific names.
Plant part	Different plant parts, organized in a hierarchical structure (with different detail levels), e.g. aerial part > leaf > young leaf.
Preparation	Different preparation steps, organized in a hierarchical structure (with different detail levels), e.g. cooked > boiled, fried.
Reliability	Sure, nearly sure, probable, presumed, doubtful, wrong.
Site	Different sites, organized in a hierarchical structure (at different spatial scales), e.g. Mediterranean > Italy > South Italy > Campania > Napoli.
Source	Source description, can be of different types (bibliographic reference, collector, informant, herbal, archeological). According to the referencing tables, only subsets of this table can be selected.
Spatial relevance	Point, local, municipality, region, province, nation.
Taxonomic level	Family, genus, species, subspecies.
Use	Different plant uses, organized in a hierarchical structure (with different detail levels), including medicinal (e.g. health > neurological disease > headache), ceremonial, alimentary, domestic and veterinary uses.
Use category	Ancient medicine, official medicine, popular, ceremonial

The archive currently allows the storage and management of following information:

- Ethnobotanical information from interviews (informants), historical herbarium specimens and documents (recent, historic and ancient sources), according to a hierarchical catalogue of plant uses and preparations (medicinal, alimentary, ceremonial, veterinary, domestic). It is also possible to include ethnobotanical information from archeological remains, although the relationships to the relative databases have not yet been implemented.

- Plant names information: plant popular names (local or ancient), and their relationship to species taxonomy. Information on reliability of species identification (also multiple options are possible, according to hypothesis of different authors);
- Information on specimens in historical herbals.

Ethnobotanical data were organized in a relational structure: a relevée can group information on multiple plants, which can be used for different scopes, each being reached with one or a sequence of preparation steps. Traditional knowledge cannot be easily categorized and therapeutic uses are often intermingled with ceremonial and symbolic ones. Since attempts to categorize these kinds of uses are not always meaningful, the storage of a description that reports in detail a specific application of a plant is recommended. However, to allow a more effective search within the database, beliefs and practices dealing with folk uses of a species were grouped in use categories, ranging over medicinal (including affection and mode of administration of the plant), ceremonial (symbolic, ritual, religious including any belief concerning the plant), alimentary, domestic (from the control of undesired animal in the house, to house construction, or wooden utensils), veterinary uses.

These categories have been organized in a hierarchical structure and may be assigned according to the detail level of the information gathered. A reliability degree of those use assignments is given, particularly for data from the ancient treatises and from archeological remains. The principle of storing information with different levels of accuracy has been implemented also for the preparation steps (mechanical breaking, cooking, drying, ...) and for the plant parts involved (above ground part, bark, leaf, young leaf, below ground part, root, bulb, tuber, ...).

This level of semantic detail allows fine tuned query possibilities and is needed if a future improvement to a multilingual application is planned.

The database is intended to store and manage data from pre-Linnean times to present. At the moment the oldest entries stored in the database, dealing with plant uses in Mediterranean region during Antiquity, come from studies carried out in the last decade on *Corpus Hippocraticum* treatises, Dioscorides "*De Materia Medica*", Pliny's *Naturalis Historia*, and Pseudo-Apuleius *Herbarium*. Since ancient texts provides no iconography and limited description of plants; the identity of these species is always a matter of controversial. For example, according to Buenz, the identification of the plants quoted in the *Corpus Hippocraticum* is a largely overcome challenge, whereas Raven is clearly skeptical about the possibility of resolving the identity of any Greek phytonym down to the species level, in accordance with Linnaean nomenclature. In order to explicitly implement in our database this uncertainty, a join table with the putative identifications of ancient phytonyms with one or more Mediterranean species has been implemented with the proposed identifications according to Aliotta et al. and Stirling. Thus this allows a critical evaluation of ancient traditional knowledge about the uses of a plant. We used this specific structure to enable us also to manage synonym relationships of scientific names or identical phythonyms referring to different species, according to regions or authors. In this respect, our phythonym table contains popular, ancient, Italian and scientific names, allowing a maximum flexibility when entering new ethnobotanical records.

Since a consistent number of our entries come from plant labels in historical herbals, also detailed information on specimen and herbal collections was stored in the database.

Information sources can be of multiple types, namely bibliographic references, collectors, informants, historical herbals or archeological remains. All or subsets of these types can be referenced, according to the tables where a source information is needed.

As already mentioned, reliability of the information stored in the database is handled at multiple levels, namely: phytonym identification (Plant table), which in the case of informants or collectors is useful, tentative identifications (Taxon assignment table), used mainly for data from the ancient treatises, and use assignments (Plant use table), for data from ancient sources or archeological remains.

Different query features allow the user to get a temporal drawing of the importance of a species within the life of a community. A query for a species or a genus returns all the available information, either from published works, unpublished interviews, labels of historical herbals or archeological remains. The hierarchical features implemented for uses, plant parts, preparations and sites (from national to municipality level) allows both generic or fine-grained queries for those parameters, according to the requirements of the user. Particular query settings can be specified, in order to extend the queries to rougher levels of detail, e.g. querying for a genus instead of a species, thus including all the species of that genus, or querying for neurology instead of headache, thus including all neurological affections. Such latter use comparisons can only be performed in the frame of the specified hierarchical structure, which implicitly defines the degree of similarity of the uses. In the future, different hierarchical classifications of the stored uses could be defined and added to the use table, thus enhancing comparative capabilities of the archive.

The performed queries return the appropriate reliability information. This is particularly important for the case of multiple putative identifications of ancient phytonyms, where a query for a given use produces multiple report lines for the same ethnobotanical information, according to the taxon assignments. The tuning of reliability settings allows restricting the query from all the record combinations (for a case by case analysis) to only records with a certain reliability degree or to only record combinations with the highest reliability.

Also historical summary information can be retrieved (analyzing the highest reliabilities), matching a plant binomial with a specific use, and showing for example how many times a given medicinal use of a species is reported in the database for a defined period.

The repository has been implemented with PostgreSQL8.3, while entry masks have been developed with Microsoft® Access 2000.

CAMPANIA AS A CASE STUDY

At present time only data on flowering plants have been stored in the database, but it is possible to extend the archive also to non-vascular plants, algae and fungi. The interval of time was chosen because plant nomenclature from XVIII century onward is based on Linnean classification, which allows a more reliable approach to species identification.

At the moment, all the data from modern (1950 – present days) ethnobotanical studies carried out in Campania have been stored in the database, together with the available information from different historical sources dating back from the first half of 1900's to XIX century. The majority of the records were extracted from hundreds of published works, both popular and scientific, which belong to three main types of sources:

(I) floristic description of a territory, which often contained ethnobotanical information (i.e. Gussone; Pasquale; Pasquale and Pasquale).

(II) the labels of the historical herbaria samples of Herbarium Porticense (PORUN), that in same case reported some indications about the use of a plant in the site where it was collected (collection Vincenzo and Francesco Briganti of Herbarium Porticense – PORUN)

(III) medical treatises of physicians of past centuries (i.e. Petagna; Limoncelli; Pasquale and Avellino), which contains also the description of folk remedies, thus representing an important source of ethnopharmacological information.

RESULTS AND DISCUSSION

Data since the XVIII century

The database currently includes 474 different species, which have been used in Campania between the end of XVIII century and the 2007.

1672 different uses have been recorded for the species listed in the database, ranging from medicinal, to alimentary, ceremonial, domestic and veterinary. Table below represents the distribution of the number of data (including number of sources of information and number of species) between XIX and XX Century.

It is not surprising that the majority of data are related to recent studies, since previously folk knowledge was often largely disregarded. Caution should be adopted to the approach of such heterogeneous material. The studies dealing with the traditional plant knowledge in Campania which have been conducted approximately from 1950s onward, have been carried out according to the procedures adopted worldwide for ethnobotanical research.

On the other hand, historical data stored in the archive allow to elicit information from sources which hardly represent a random sample of a statistic population.

They can be derived from a single observation or from memories of very few individuals, and are only rarely a detailed recollection of uses coming from a population.

The structure of information on plant uses from past centuries precludes any quantitative approach in comparison between past and present traditional knowledge of populations living in Campania. Notwithstanding this limitation, the historical ethnobotanical archive represents a useful tool to understand cultural transformations occurring on plant uses over the generations, particularly shedding light on continuity and changes in folk phytotherapy.

Table: Number of Campanian ethnobotanical records of plants in the last two century, according to the stored datasets.

Time (period)	Number of data	Number of information sources	Number of species
2000–2007	333426 *	4	162238 *
1950–1999	645242 *	27	282138 *
1900–1949	103	13	60
1850–1899	150	9	120
1800–1849	59	9	49
Total	1958	62	558

Numbers are referred to published data; * number of unpublished data.

From the analysis of the information stored in the database, it is possible to make some generalizations on the evolution of ethnobotanical knowledge in Campania. Several trends remain unchanged over the last two centuries, such as the prevalence of data about medicinal plants, included those used in the so-called food medicine, which was often mentioned in XIX century sources. The occurrence of a relatively high number of medicinal citations is also due to the interests of the authors of that time, generally physicians or chemists.

The data were analyzed for both content and geographical distribution.

Table below lists the plants already employed in Campania at the beginning of XIX Century, which are still in use. Some species have been used for multiple purposes, including those related to food, medicine, ceremonies, and magic rituals. According to Turner, "the more widely or intensively a plant is used, the greater its cultural significance". If we take this assumption as a general rule, it is possible to derive from Table below a rank of significance for each plant included, although in a preliminary and qualitative way. In this respect, it is not surprising that the cultural importance of some species as *Olea europea* L. and *Vitis vinifera* L., followed by *Brassica oleracea* L. ranked highest in usage, and consequently in cultural significance, in the Campanian territory. The domestication and cultivation of these species was of pivotal importance in the Mediterranean civilization since Neolithic times, and represent still now an important economic resource for the Campania and the whole Mediterranean Region.

The treatment of a range of internal affections with the so called food medicine often relies upon cultivated plants; in general, the collection of wild greens, although still practiced, has been considerably reduced in present times. This is probably due to the continuous decrease of people able to recognize plants in the wild, which, in turn, has been determined by the decline of agriculture in the region. However, cultivated plants correspond to about 30% of the species recorded in Table below, the remaining being wild species, and it is possible to infer some degree of significance also for these species. For a detailed comparison, we selected three wild gathered species, *Adiantum capillus-veneris* L., *Parietaria judaica* L., and *Artemisia absinthium* L. frequently used in Campania.

Table: Plants used in Campanian folk therapy at the beginning of XIX Century, which are still in use.

Species	Medicinal	Food	Domestic	Ceremonial	Veterinary
Adiantum capillus-veneris L.	•				
Ajuga reptans L.	•				
Allium cepa L. *	•	•			
Allium sativum L. *	•	•		•	
Apium graveolens L.		•			
Apium nodiflorum (L.) Lag.		•			
Artemisia absinthium L.	•			•	
Asparagus acutifolius L.		•			
Asparagus officinalis L. *	•	•			
Brassica oleracea L. *	•	•			•
Brassica rapa L. s.l. *	•	•			
Chamaerops humilis L. *			•	•	
Cichorium intybus L. s.l.	•	•			

Clematis flammula L.		•			•
Clematis vitalba L.		•			
Castanea sativa Mill. *		•	•		
Colchicum autumnale L. *	•	•			
Conium maculatum L.	•				
Cyclamen hederifolium Aiton	•				•
Cydonia oblonga Mill. *	•	•			
Cynodon dactylon (L.) Pers.					•
Datura stramonium L. S.l.	•				
Dianthus sp.	•				
Diplotaxis tenuifolia (L.) DC.	•	•			
Erica arborea L.			•	•	
Euonymus europaeus L.	•				
Euphorbia helioscopia L. s.l.	•				
Festuca arundinacea Schreb. subsp. *corsica* (Hoek.) Kerguélen		•			
Fragaria vesca L. s.l.	•	•			
Fraxinus ornus L. s.l.	•				
Fumaria capreolata L. s.l.	•	•			
Fumaria officinalis L. s.l.	•	•			
Hordeum vulgare L. *	•	•			
Juglans regia L. *	•	•	•	•	•
Lactuca sativa L. *	•	•			
Lavandula angustifolia Mill. s.l.	•		•		
Malus domestica (Borkh.) Borkh. *	•	•			
Matricaria chamomilla L.	•				
Mentha sp.	•	•			
Mentha × *piperita* L. *	•	•			
Nerium oleander L. s.l. *	•				
Olea europaea L. *	•	•		•	
Origanum majorana L. *	•	•			
Origanum vulgare L. S.l.	•	•			
Papaver rhoeas L. s.l.	•				
Parietaria judaica L.	•	•			
Persicaria hydropiper (L.) Delarbre	•	•			
Petroselinum crispum (Mill.) Fuss *	•	•			
Pimpinella anisum L. *	•	•			
Plantago major L. s.l.	•				

Portulaca oleracea L. s.l.		•			
Quercus sp.	•				
Rubus sp.	•	•		•	
Ruscus aculeatus L.	•	•	•	•	•
Ruta sp.	•				
Ruta graveolens L. *	•				
Salix alba L.	•				
Sambucus nigra L.	•	•			
Sanguisorba minor Scop. s.l.		•			
Sedum telephium L. s.l.	•				
Sonchus oleraceus L.		•			
Sonchus tenerrimus L.		•			
Stellaria media (L.) Vill. s.l.	•				
Teucrium chamaedrys L. s.l.	•				
Trifolium incarnatum L. s.l.					•
Triticum aestivum L. *	•	•			
Typha latifolia L.			•		
Verbena sp.	•				
Verbena officinalis L.	•				
Vitis vinifera L. *	•	•	•		•

(*) Cultivated plants.

It is evident that even though the general significance of these plants, based on the number of usages, remained unmodified, many present uses differ from those of XIX Century. The analysis of data suggests that in XIX, and in the first decade of the following Century, the selected plants were primarily used as pain-killer, and as febrifuge, whercas their reliance for these scopes is now less frequently reported.

The capillary spread of conventional pharmaceuticals products, comparatively safer and more efficacious, has probably caused the disappearance of this medicinal use. On the other hand, some new applications probably borrowed from health public media, have been introduced, as indicated by the application of some plants against metabolic diseases, such as high blood pressure, and hypercholesterolemia.

Table: Campanian ethnopharmacological uses of **Adiantum capillus-veneris** *L.*, **Artemisia absinthium** *L. and* **Parietaria judaica** *L. in the last two centuries.*

Campanian ethnopharmacological uses of *Adiantum capillus-veneris* L., *Artemisia absinthium* L. and *Parietaria judaica* L. in the last two centuries.

Botanical name	Uses description	Part used	Preparations
Adiantum capillus-veneris L.	Against labour pains	Aerial part	Decoction
	Emmenagogue	Aerial part	Infusion
	Local application on sores	Leaves	External use
	Respiratory system affections: emollient, expectorant	Aerial part	Infusion
	Resolvent for contusions, antiecchymotic	Aerial part	Decoction
	Antitussive, for sore-throat and loss of speech. Externally against hair loss and dandruff	Aerial part	Infusion
	Abortive, regulator of menses, anti-cough	Aerial part	Decoction of leaves with some dried figs, an apple, some *Prunus cerasus* L. fruits, some pieces of *Prunus dulcis* (Mill.) D.A. Webb epicarpus
	Expectorant, antitussive, in the treatment of bronchitis, against dandruff and seborrhea	Aerial part	Decoction, infusion and tincture
	Antihelmintic	Aerial part	Decoction

EXTENSION OF THE TEMPORAL CONTEXT TO THE ANTIQUITY

The Campanian historical database encompasses also information on plant uses in ancient Mediterranen cultures, particularly of Greek and Roman phytotherapy.

This inclusion needs some methodological considerations: in a straightforward assay, the anthropologist Di Nola categorized different kinds of ethnomedicine.

The first one fits the Hoppal definition: "ethnomedicine is the term for the practice of folk healing in the recent ethnographic literature".

This definition embraces not only the study of cultures lacking written traditions, but also the body of traditional knowledge of European rural communities.

According to Di Nola also the corpus of knowledge belonging to the Ancient Classic medicine can be considered as a sort of ethnomedicine.

It consists of treatises where popular phyto-remedies are described, although often tightly intermingled with a scholar approach to the therapy of some diseases.

It cannot be denied that a thread linking Ancient and contemporary ethnobotany in Mediterranean Countries can be ideally traced: Stannard stressed that not few curative practices elaborated in early times of Western civilization had remained alive.

On the other hand, the caution evoked for the evaluation of ethnobotanical data coming from the last two centuries must be multiplied when one aims to analyze different uses of plants over a so large temporal period.

Paul suggested that popular therapeutics is prevalently made by old medical prescriptions, which were subsequently abandoned by official Medicine.

To shed light on this point, the medicinal uses of *A. capillus-veneris*, *A. absinthium* and *P. judaica* have been reported in tablebelow, according to some of the most important medical treatises of Antiquity and to a medical text of XVIII Century written by V. Petagna.

In this way, it is possible to trace the possible influence on present popular medicine of historical recipes from different periods.

As can be seen, during Antiquity *A. capillus-veneris* was administred mainly against pulmonar and kidney affections, and to treat gynecological diseases, *A. absinthium* was highly reputed as a tonic and digestive, and as a powerful antiworming agent and *P. judaica* had application as a diuretic, in the therapy of skin affections and to help the resolution of traumatic accidents.

Similar therapeutic uses are also descripted by Petagna. A comparison with the present ethnopharmacological knowledge in Campania indicate that only some of the oldest applications are still in use, and that, as expected, there are more similarities between the indications reported by Petagna and the present uses of the selected plants.

However, no general rule can be traced; the story of uses of each plant follows hardly identifiable trajectories, which need a detailed study of all available sources.

A point break is the transition from Antiquity to the Christian Era, when new symbolic meanings were introduced for many plants, renforcing old therapeutical applications or also relating them to unexplored medical applications, as in the case of *Rosmarinus officinalis* in Latin America.

In this respect, the comparison of the TK of a restricted territory as that of Campania with the corpus of Ancient phytotherapy can not be exhaustive and needs a more detailed scrutiny carried out on a larger set of historical data from other territories of the Mediterranean region.

Table: Campanian ethnopharmacological uses of **Adiantum capillus-veneris** *L.*, **Artemisia absinthium** *L. and* **Parietaria judaica** *L. in medical treatises writttten in different historical periods.*

	Affection	Part(s) of plant	Preparation
Adiantum capillus-veneris L.			
Corpus Hippocraticum	diuretic	aerial part	decoction
	jaundice	aerial part	potion
	to promote menses	aerial part	potion
	uterine affection	aerial part	potion
	against leucorrhaea	aerial part	potion with wine
	rectum prolapsus	aerial part	local application
	to relieve partum complaints	aerial part	potion
	to easy placenta expulsion	aerial part	potion
	to facilitate the conception	aerial part	local fumigation
Dioscorides	against asthma	aerial part	decoction
	jaundice	aerial part	decoction
	mycosis	aerial part	decoction
	lithiasis and related affections	aerial part	decoction
	against diarrhoea	aerial part	decoction
	gynecological affections	aerial part	potion with wine
	emmenagogue	aerial part	potion with wine
	against hair losses	aerial part	local application, also in mixture with laudanum, hyssop and honey

	against alopaecia	aerial part	local application
	skin affections	aerial part	local application
Pliny	affections of the liver and spleen	aerial part	decoction
	against asthma	aerial part	decoction
	against excoriations of infants	aerial part	liniment combined with rose-oil, local application
	against head-ache	aerial part	local application
	antidote to the venom of serpents and spiders	aerial part	local application
	anti-hæmorrhagic	aerial part	potion with vinegar
	calculi of the bladder	aerial part	potion
	diuretic	aerial part	potion with wine
	expulsion of after-birth, emmenagogue	aerial part	potion
	looseness of the bowels	aerial part	decoction in wine
	skin affections	aerial part	local application
	strangury and affections of the kidneys	aerial part	liniment, local application
Pseudo Apuleius	abdominal pain	leaves	wine potion with coriander and pepper seeds
Petagna	respiratory system affections	aerial part	infusion, sirup
Corpus Hippocraticum	against sterility	aerial part	not described
	emmenagogue	aerial part	local application, macerated in white wine
	jaundice	aerial part	not described

	opistotonus (neck rigidity)	aerial part	not described
	post partum affections	aerial part	infusion
	uterine affections	aerial part	local application
Dioscorides	against animal bites or poisonous plants	aerial part	wine potion
	against mosquito bites	aerial part	poultice mixed with oil
	dropsy and spleen pains	aerial part	poultice with Cyprus ointment
	ear and tooth pains	aerial part	decoction
	eye affections	aerial part	local application: the plant mixed with oil or honey
	jaundice, inappetence	aerial part	decoction
	sore throat	aerial part	ointment with figs soda and rye-grass flour
	stomach and visceral pains	aerial part	poultice (topic application) or potion
	tonic	aerial part	wine potion
Pliny	antidote to animal and plant poisons	aerial part	potion with vinegar or wine
	antihelmintic	aerial part	potion of the extracted juice
	diuretic	aerial part	potion with gallic nard
	ear affections	aerial part	decoction, local application or liniment of the plant bruised with honey
	emmenagogue	aerial part	taken with honey or employed as a pessary
	eye affections	aerial part	local application, with raisin wine or honey

	jaundice	aerial part	eaten raw, with parsley or adiantum
	liver complaints	aerial part	potion with gallic nard
	iliac regions affection	aerial part	plaster with Cyprian wax or figs
	purgative	seeds	potion with sea water and honey
	sea sickness	aerial part	potion drunken as a preventive
	skin affections	aerial part	water infusion
	spleen diseases	aerial part	potion with vinegar and figs
	stomach affections	aerial part	decoction, or raw with rue, pepper, and salt
	to dispel nausea and flatulency	aerial part	potion with the addition of sile, gallic narde and a little vinegar
	tonic	aerial part	decoction
	wounds	aerial part	local application
Pseudo Apuleius	not reported	——	——
Petagna	hypochondria, hysteria	leaves	extract through the soap
	To stimulate liver function	leaves	extract through the soap
	against malaria	——	1/2 spoon of juice of the plant with clove in wine
	against scurvy	leaves	infusion
	against dropsy	leaves	infusion
	antihelmintic	leaves	1 spoon of essence
	headache		Powdered leaves mixed with sugar, or infusion of diluted wine

	eyes inflammation		powder of leaves mixed with sugar, or infusion of diluted wine
	edemata	leaves	fresh leaves
	gangrene	leaves	boiled in the sea water
Corpus Hippocraticum	abortive	leaves	potion
Dioscorides	skin affection	leaves	local application
	glandular inflammation	leaves	local application
	oedema	leaves	local application
	ulcerations	leaves	juice and white lead ointment
	sore throat	leaves	ointment or juice gargle
	earache	leaves	ointment with rose oil
	cough	leaves	juice
Pliny	for suppurated abscesses	leaves	the juice taken warm
	to cure convulsions	leaves	the juice taken warm
	to cure ruptures, bruises	leaves	the juice taken warm
Pseudo Apuleius	gout	aerial part	decoction mixed with pork fat and applied on foots or knee
Petagna	emollient	leaves	juice, decoction with bearberry
	resolvent	leaves	juice, decoction with bearberry
	diuretic	leaves	juice, decoction with bearberry

The black dots indicate the same medicinal aims use while the white dots similar use.

CONCLUSION

The Mediterranean region, with its complex history, still needs historical studies dealing on traditional knowledge of plants. This database revealed to be a useful tool to store and to compare present and previous ethnobotanical uses in the Campanian region. The collection of data is in progress. Further information could be gathered in small libraries and local archives present almost in an Campanian towns, where it could be possible to find forgotten sources dealing with local traditions.

In the next future it is necessary to finalize the structure of the database for publishing it online, adding multilingual support and administration of user privileges, in order to be contributed by other researchers, thus enhancing the Mediterranean ethnobotanical network.

11

Plants and Traditional Knowledge: an Ethnobotanical Investigation

BACKGROUND

Documenting and safeguarding Traditional Ecological Knowledge (TEK) have become central issues in the planning and management of natural resources. Traditional knowledge of plants and their uses is the result of thousands of years of experience (both apprenticeship and self-directed learning-while-doing) and educational methods (e.g. telling stories). The relevance of this knowledge as far as increasing the daily living standards of rural populations is concerned, as well as in taking decisions regarding the sustainable use of plant resources, has frequently been noted.

However, in developed countries, this traditional knowledge is being widely threatened by current trends of economic globalization that promote intensive agriculture, industrialization, and the migration of rural populations to urban areas. Consequently, it is crucial to record this fast-disappearing knowledge before it vanishes definitively along with the present generation of elderly persons.

Due to its geographic isolation, the island of Sardinia (Italy) has been exposed to very few external influences, and up until now this has promoted a very high cultural homogeneity and stability. In Sardinia, people are still very proud of their traditional cultural heritage, and a lot of "folk" uses of plants are still maintained, especially in rural and mountain areas.

The aim of this study is to record local knowledge regarding plants and their traditional uses and to assess how this knowledge is distributed within a community of central Sardinia (Italy) situated in the area of Barbagia, one of the richest areas as far as ancient popular traditions are concerned.

The study area, which is located to the west of the town of Nuoro (40°19'16" N, 3°04'05" W) in central Sardinia, is approximately 40 sq km wide. Monte Ortobene is a mountain whose altitudes range up to 995 m. Due to its proximity to the city (approximately 8 km) and easy access, it is one of the areas most frequented by the local community. Only a few natives still live on Monte Ortobene, while many people come here from the nearby city of Nuoro for the purposes of recreational hiking. The economy of the Nuoro municipality, which is the largest populated center in Barbagia, is based mainly on agriculture, handicrafts, and tourism. The population of the entire municipality reaches approximately 36,000 inhabitants (164,000 in the province of Nuoro), with a density of 190.73 inhabitants per sq km. The climate is typically Mediterranean, with rainfall concentrated during the autumn and winter and hot, very dry summers. The prevailing geological substrate is granite. The local vegetation consists mainly of different stages of Mediterranean series (maquis, scrubs, grasslands). The first definite evidence of human settlement in this area dates from 3800 B.C. to 2800 B.C, as attested by the presence of collective hypogeous graves called *Domus de Janas* ('Fairy houses').

Methods

The investigation was carried out from 2004 to 2005. Information was collected on traditional uses of wild plants and also of cultivated ones; however, in the latter case, only uses different from those for which each plant is commonly grown were considered (e. g. using wheat to decorate altars). Uses concerning materials derived from plants but thoroughly processed (e.g. vinegar, bread) were not recorded. Special care was taken in choosing the informants. Only people who were born and had always lived in the area were taken into consideration, and we also made sure that the source of their knowledge about local uses of plants had only been a question of traditional culture. Due to these strict criteria, only 17 informants were selected and involved in the study. Information was collected by means of semi-structured interviews, because when the informants were interviewed, the detailed prearranged questionnaires proved to be too rigid. The interviews were characterized by empathy and confidence with the informants, together with an attitude of listening and respect, on the part of the interviewer.

Voucher specimens of the cited plant species were prepared and deposited in the FIAF (University of Florence, Erbario dei laboratori di Botanica Agraria e forestale) herbarium. Systematic arrangement and nomenclature mostly followed Pignatti's Flora d'Italia. In a few instances of plants belonging to critical groups (e.g.: *Taraxacum officinale* Weber), we resorted to a broad concept of the species (species *sensu lato*), as this appeared to be more suitable when dealing with ethnobotanical data.

All the collected data were filed in a data-base (*analytical table*) consisting of a spreadsheet (Windows Excel 2003). The rows on it corresponded to the species reported, and the columns contained information on each species. As discussed in a previous contribution, each row in the analytical table represents an elementary record and is intended as a *citation*, i.e. a single use reported for a single species by a single informant. Each citation is supplemented by the following data (see below for explanations):

- Scientific name (species or subspecies)
- Botanical family
- Local vernacular name(s)
- Part(s) of the plant used
- Category of use (i.e. general typology)
- Secondary category of use (i.e. detailed typology)
- Way of use
- Whether the plant is wild or cultivated

- Local frequency
- Habitat
- Notes

For medicinal plants, further information was also recorded.

Apart from scientific names and classification, all the data were reported just as they had been related by the informants.

Category of use is defined as one of the following general typologies of use (for categories marked with an *, no use was reported in this investigation):

- Agropastoral
- Alimentary
- Domestic
- Drugs and cigarettes*
- Handicrafts
- Hunting and fishing*
- Ludic
- Magical/medicinal
- Magical/Ritual/Propitiatory
- Medicinal
- Religious
- Veterinary*

Note that many uses pertaining to all categories included some magical aspect, but only those in which a magical element was predominant were included in the 'Magical/Ritual/Propitiatory' category. Furthermore, uses were included in the handicrafts category only if the material involved was processed or converted in appreciable ways and the product is durable.

Secondary category of use is intended as a detailed typology identified within each category. In filing and processing data, secondary category of use was assumed to be the most detailed level in discriminating different uses from one another. For medicinal plants, secondary categories coincided with general therapeutic indications, such as dermatological affections, diseases of the digestive system, etc. Moreover, since uses in this category are more complex and articulate, additional information has been provided: detailed therapeutic indications (e.g. gastritis, nausea, etc.), way of preparation, and way of administration. Olive oil was taken into consideration as a phytoterapeutic remedy only when it was considered by the informant to be an effective component of the medicament, and not merely a solvent or medium, as was the case for ointments or macerations in oil.

Way of use is a short description of how the plant is used: preparation, recipes, etc.

In *Notes*, possible further information is reported, such as proverbs, toponyms, notes on past frequency, etc.

We considered as distinct citations those differing from one another in at least one of the following data: species, informant, secondary category of use. Citations differing in minor aspects, such as the part of the plant used, the way of use, and (in medicinal uses) detailed therapeutic indication, way of preparation, and the way of administration were combined into a single citation. Each citation coincides with a single row in the analytical table.

The number of *uses* was obtained by considering as distinct uses for each species those differing in secondary category. Therefore, citations reported for the same secondary category by different informants were counted only once.

We applied quantitative analysis of the data through the use of certain synthetic indexes. Despite the fact that we collected information from only a small number of informants, we tested this quantitative approach in order to verify whether it could improve understanding and interpretation of the results of our investigation. We intended to assess whether synthetic indexes could help to quantify the distribution and diversity of information in each species of plant and/or in each informant, and also the different relevance of each botanical species, even while dealing with very few data. The following synthetic indexes were used:

Local importance of each species was calculated by using the Relative Frequency of Citation (RFC):

$$RFC = \frac{FC}{N}$$

where FC is the number of informants who mentioned the use of the species and N is the total number of informants (17 in this study).

Diversity of information within each species was calculated using two different indexes: The Cultural Importance Index (CI_s), calculated by using the formula suggested in:

$$CI_S = \sum_{u=u_1}^{u_{NC}} \sum_{i=i_1}^{i_N} UR_{ui} / N$$

where u is the category of use, NC is the total number of different categories of use (of each 'i' species), UR is the total number of use-reports for each species (corresponding in the present study to 'citations' as defined above), and N is the total number of informants (17 in this study). In calculating NC, defined in as the 'total number of use-categories', for each species we considered the number of different 'secondary categories of use' as defined above. However, it must be noted that these were much more detailed and numerous than the 'use-categories' adopted.

The Shannon-Wiener Index (H'), calculated by using the formula:

$$H' = -\sum_{i=1}^{u} (pi)(\log pi) \text{ base } 10$$

where u is the number of uses and

$$pi = n_i / N, N = \sum_{i=1}^{u} n$$

where n_i is the number of citations for each use (as explained previously, a citation is a single use reported for a single species by a single informant) and N is the total number of citations. This index has been widely employed in order to quantify knowledge distribution in different communities. Here, however, it should be noted that it is applied to a diversity of uses, both within each species and between different species.

Evenness was calculated with the Evenness Index (J), using the formula:

$$J = \frac{H'}{\log UR_{ui}}$$

where H' is the Shannon-Wiener Index and UR_{ui} is the number of uses reported for each species.

RESULTS AND DISCUSSION

Informants

As pointed out above, only 17 informants were interviewed: three men (17.6%) and 14 women (82.4%). This uneven repartition is not unusual in ethnobotanical investigations in Italy (see, for instance, as a consequence of the importance of women in the domestic context, which is where most plant resources, especially alimentary and medicinal plants, are managed.

This also means that, in the current investigation, women proved to be the main upholders of traditions linked to domestic life. Only one informant (5.9%) was younger than 60; 10 (58.8%) were 61–75 years old, and 6 (35.3%) were over 65.

Most of them (15, i.e. 88.2%) were retired; only two (11.8%) were still working.

Women worked mostly as housewives (8, i.e. 47.1% of all the informants). As for educational qualifications, 9 (52.9%) had had only a primary-school ('scuola elementare') education; one (5.9%), a grammar-school ('scuola media') education; 6 (35.3%) a high-school ('scuola superiore') education; and only one (5.9%) had a university degree. See Table below for summarized information on the informants.

Table: Informants – Demographic data

	n	%
Age		
Under 60	1	*5.9*
61–75	10	*58.8*
Above 75	6	*35.3*
Sex		
Men	3	*17.6*
Women	14	*82.4*
Education		
Primary school	9	*52.9*
Secondary school	1	*5.9*
High school	6	*35.3*
University degree	1	*5.9*
Occupation		
Housewives	8	*47.1*
Employees	5	*29.4*
Hospital nurses	3	*17.6*
Others	1	*5.9*
Retired	15	*88.2*
Employed	2	*11.8*

PLANTS. GENERAL CONSIDERATIONS

The main results on informants, plants and uses are reported in several synthetic tables.

Table: Ethnobotanical plants – Synthesis of main results

Number of species	99
Number of citations	301
Number of uses	191
Number of different secondary categories of use	50

Table: Ethnobotanical plants – Categories of use

Category	Number of citations	Number of species	Number of uses (secondary categories)
Alimentary	126	44	13
Medicinal	106	40	12
Domestic	23	15	8
Ludic	21	15	5
Agropastoral	8	7	5
Magic/Medicinal	6	5	2
Religious	7	4	1
Handicraft	2	2	2
Magic/ritual/propitiatory	2	2	2

Table: Ethnobotanical plants – Botanical families

Compositae	22	57
Liliaceae	7	36
Rosaceae	7	24
Umbelliferae	6	19
Malvaceae	4	27
Labiatae	4	10
Urticaceae	4	9
Leguminosae	4	8
Graminaceae	4	7
Cruciferae	4	6
Apocynaceae	3	5
Cistaceae	3	3
Oleaceae	2	9
Myrtaceae	2	5
Plantaginaceae	2	4
Boraginaceae	2	4
Crassulaceae	2	4
Chenopodiaceae	1	16
Cactaceae	1	9
Ericaceae	1	7
Lauraceae	1	5

Araliaceae	1	4
Fagaceae	1	3
Guttiferae	1	3
Polygonaceae	1	3
Anacardiaceae	1	3
Papaveraceae	1	2
Juncaceae	1	2
Pinaceae	1	2
Euphorbiaceae	1	1
Ranunculaceae	1	1
Scrophulariaceae	1	1
Caprifoliaceae	1	1
Palmae	1	1

Table: Ethnobotanical plants – Wild/cultivated

	Number of Species
Wild	89
Cultivated	6
Wild and cultivated	3
Not present in the area	1

Table: Ethnobotanical plants – Knowledge distribution

	Number of species
Mentioned by 12 informants	1
Mentioned by 11 informants	0
Mentioned by 10 informants	0
Mentioned by 9 informants	1
Mentioned by 8 informants	0
Mentioned by 7 informants	2
Mentioned by 6 informants	0
Mentioned by 5 informants	1
Mentioned by 4 informants	8
Mentioned by 3 informants	9
Mentioned by 2 informants	23
Mentioned by 1 informant	54

Table: Ethnobotanical plants – Most mentioned species

Species	*Informants mentioning the species*
Asparagus acutifolius L.	12
Beta vulgaris L.	9
Malva sylvestris L.	7
Opuntia ficus-indica (L.) Miller	7
Olea europaea L. var. *europaea*	5
Arbutus unedo L.	4
Cichorium intybus L.	4
Ferula communis L.	4
Foeniculum vulgare Miller subsp. *piperitum* (Ucria) Coutinho	4
Laurus nobilis L.	4
Mentha suaveolens Ehrh. subsp. *insularis* (Req.) Greuter	4
Parietaria diffusa M. et K.	4
Rubus ulmifolius Schott	4

Table: Ethnobotanical plants – More versatile species

species	**number of secondary categories**	**number of categories**
Asparagus acutifolius L.	6	5
Arbutus unedo L.	5	4
Malva sylvestris L.	9	3
Opuntia ficus-indica (L.) Miller	4	3
Cydonia oblonga Miller	3	3
Olea europaea L. var. *sylvestris* Brot.	3	3
Rubus ulmifolius Schott	6	2
Cichorium intybus L.	5	2
Crataegus monogyna Jacq.	4	2
Taraxacum officinale Weber (s. l.)	4	2
Lavatera cretica L.	6	1
Matricaria chamomilla L.	5	1

Table: Ethnobotanical plants – Local frequency of species

	Number of species	%
Very common	53	*53,5*
Moderately common	36	*36,4*
Rare	9	*9,1*
Not present in the area	1	*1,0*

Table: Ethnobotanical plants – Habitats

	Number of species	%
Wastelands, marginal areas, courtyards, roadsides	58	58.6
Garrigues and shrubs	17	17.2
Wet and shady sites, near streams	14	14.1
Field edges, fences and hedges, dry walls	8	8.1
Cultivated landas, olive groves	8	8.1
Woods and maquis	6	6.1
Nearly everywhere	5	5.1
Mountain meadows	3	3
Rocks and rocky soils	3	3
North-facing mountainside	2	2
South-facing mountainside	1	1
Not present in the area	1	1

A total of 72 different plants were cited by the informants as being traditionally used in the area. These corresponded to 72 *ethnospecies*. With approximately the same meaning, Berlin suggests the use of the term *folk generic*; other authors, however, use different terms (see, for instance, Atran's *generic species*). Based on a botanical identification of the specimens, these 72 ethnospecies correspond to 99 taxa (species or, in a few cases, subspecies) belonging to 83 genera and 34 families. Sixty-nine ethnospecies were identified by the informants with specific local names; three (corresponding to the botanical species *Plantago coronopus*, *Plantago lanceolata* and *Sanguisorba minor*) were recognized by the informants as a single ethnospecies, but no folk names were recorded. The rate of correspondence between folk names and scientific names was 81%. Nineteen percent of the folk names showed *under differentiation*: i.e. a single ethnospecies name was used to indicate more than one botanical species (or subspecies) that sometimes even belonged to different botanical genera and families. The families most mentioned by the informants were Compositae (22 species, 57 citations), Liliaceae (7, 36), Rosaceae (7, 24, and Umbelliferae (6, 19). This is probably because of the abundance of these families in the Mediterranean flora, but it is also worth noting that they include many plants commonly used in Italy as food and natural medicine. Eighty-nine out of the 99 species grow wild, six are cultivated, three can be found either as wild or cultivated, and one (*Chamaerops humilis*) does not grow in the area under investigation and was usually collected in the surrounding areas.

A total of 301 citations was recorded, for 191 different uses belonging to 50 different secondary categories of use. The most relevant categories of use were Alimentary and Medicinal. Knowledge of the traditional uses of plants was heterogeneous and unevenly distributed among the informants. Average values were 11.70 species and 18.59 uses known to each informant, but 70 species and 109 uses were reported by a single key-informant. Twenty-two species were mentioned by 3 or more informants. Out of these, only one was cited by more than 10 informants. This result probably reflects the disappearance of particular knowledge, rather than a low ethnobotanical value of the species cited by only one or two informants.

The species most mentioned were *Asparagus acutiflolius* (12 informants, 27 citations), *Beta vulgaris* (9, 16), *Malva sylvestris* (7, 19), *Opuntia ficus-indica* (7, 11), and *Olea europaea* var. *europaea* (5, 6). For most species (79%), only 1 to 2 different uses were reported. Species showing the highest versatility, understood as being the highest number of different categories and secondary categories of use, were *Asparagus acutifolius* (5 different categories and 6 different secondary categories), *Arbutus unedo* (4 categories, 5 secondary categories), *Malva sylvestris* (3, 9), and *Opuntia ficus-indica* (3, 4). However, when only secondary categories of use were considered, *Rubus ulmifolius* (6 secondary categories, 2 categories), *Lavatera cretica* (6, 1),

Cichorium intybus (5, 2), and *Matricaria chamomilla* (5, 1) were also found to be highly versatile. As for the local frequency of species, 53 species out of 99 (53.5%) were defined by the informants as 'very common', 36 (36.4%) as 'moderately common' and only 9 (9.1%) as 'rare' (one species was not present in the area).

Plants of ethnobotanical interest were collected in 13 different environments. Ruderal species from wastelands, marginal areas, courtyards, and roadsides formed the largest portion (58.6%), followed by species growing in garrigues and shrubs (17.2%) and in wet and shady sites (14.1%). The predominance of the collection and consumption of species from environments marked and disturbed by human activity, rather than from less disturbed or pristine environments, is a common result in ethnobotanical studies, although few studies mention or discuss this point. Many hypotheses can be suggested as being possible explanations for this feature. First of all, people started recognizing and using wild plants that were easier to gather, such as those growing close to houses, roads, cultivated or fallow fields, and field boundaries. Many of the plants gathered in disturbed environments may also behave like weeds or opportunistic commensals in different agricultural practices, and have somehow co-evolved with the presence of man. It is also possible that some species of ethnobotanical interest were cultivated in the past and became wild afterwards. It should also be noted that only 38 (41%) out of the 92 species growing wild in the area (including 3 species that are both wild and cultivated) were mentioned in 1957 in Rovinetti's phytogeographical contribution. This can be explained in different ways. It is possible that, although he had been investigating in the area of Monte Ortobene for five years, Rovinetti failed to consider certain habitats, such as ruderal and marginal ones and ecotones, which are rich in plants of ethnobotanical interest. The possibility of floristic changes having taken place in past decades appears to be rather unlikely, since all the plants were cited as being traditionally used by old people.

Table below reports the results of quantitative analysis for the 20 most relevant and useful species in the area of Monte Ortobene.

Table: Results of quantitative analysis for the 20 most relevant species

	Basic values			Indices				Ranking		
Species	**FC**	**NC**	**UR**	**RFC**	**CI**	**H'**	**J**	**RFC**	**CI**	**H'**
Asparagus acutifolius L.	12	6	27	0.71	1.59	0.60	0.78	1	1	6
Beta vulgaris L.	9	3	16	0.53	0.94	0.38	0.79	2	3	13
Malva sylvestris L.	7	9	19	0.41	1.12	0.81	0.85	3	2	1
Opuntia ficus-indica (L.) Miller	7	4	9	0.41	0.53	0.57	0.95	4	6	7
Olea europaea L. var.*europaea*	5	3	6	0.29	0.35	0.44	0.92	5	9	11
Rubus ulmifolius Schott	4	6	10	0.24	0.59	0.76	0.98	6	5	2
Arbutus unedo L.	4	5	7	0.24	0.41	0.64	0.92	7	7	4
Cichorium intybus L.	4	5	11	0.24	0.65	0.64	0.91	8	4	5
Laurus nobilis L.	4	3	5	0.24	0.29	0.41	0.86	9	11	12
Parietaria diffusa Mert. et Koch	4	2	5	0.24	0.29	0.22	0.72	10	12	19
Ferula communis L.	4	2	5	0.24	0.29	0.22	0.72	11	13	18
Foeniculum vulgare Mill. subsp.*piperitum* (Ucria) Coutinho	4	2	7	0.24	0.41	0.30	0.99	12	8	14
Mentha suaveolens Ehrh. subsp.*insularis* (Req.) Greuter	4	2	4	0.24	0.24	0.24	0.81	13	14	17
Matricaria chamomilla L.	3	5	6	0.18	0.35	0.68	0.97	14	10	3
Hedera helix L.	3	3	4	0.18	0.24	0.45	0.95	15	15	10
Daucus carota L. subsp.*carota*	3	3	4	0.18	0.24	0.45	0.95	16	16	9
Cydonia oblonga Miller	3	3	4	0.18	0.24	0.45	0.95	17	17	8
Rumex thyrsoides Desf.	3	2	3	0.18	0.18	0.28	0.92	18	18	16
Prunus spinosa L.	3	2	3	0.18	0.18	0.28	0.92	19	19	15
Allium triquetrum L.	3	1	3	0.18	0.18	0.00	0.00	20	20	20

Basic values: FC = Number of informants mentioning the species; NC = Number of different uses ('secondary categories of use'); UR = Number of reports ('citations').Indexes: RFC = Relative Frequency of Citation; CI = Cultural Importance Index; H'= Shannon-Wiener Index; J = Evenness index. (See 'Material and methods' for further explanations).

Asparagus acutifolius was the most used species (RFC = 0.71) and the most culturally significant (CI = 1.59). *Beta vulgaris* and *Malva sylvestris* were the second most important species, but the order varied, depending on the chosen index.

The CI placed *Malva sylvestris* in second place, because it assigned a greater importance to the higher versatility of this species. On the other hand, the RFC took into consideration only the knowledge of useful plants, i.e. the number of informants who mentioned them as being useful, and *Beta vulgaris* was cited by more informants than *Malva sylvestris*.

Table above also shows that *Asparagus acutifolius* and *Beta vulgaris* reached the 6th (H' = 0.60) and 13th (H' = 0.38) places, respectively, when the diversity of knowledge and its pattern of distribution within each species were considered.

Moreover, *Rubus ulmifolius* was in 6th place when only the number of informants was taken into account, (RFC = 0.24), but rose to 5th place when the diversity of uses was considered (CI = 0.59) and to 2nd place on the basis of the Shannon-Wiener Index (H' = 0.76). The distribution of information was highly homogeneous for this species (Evenness = 0.98), and this can explain the high ranking based on the Shannon-Wiener Index.

Due to the small number of informants, the results of the quantitative analysis were not as reliable as they could have been from a statistical point of view. However, these data were both encouraging and consistent with previous studies reporting on the use of synthetic indexes. In our opinion, they could be valuable in a general discussion on the use of quantitative analysis in ethnobotanical research, and can be regarded as a pilot methodology for providing possible indications for further studies involving a larger number of informants (see, in particular, the use of the Shannon-Wiener Index to assess the diversity of uses within and between species).

In the following sections, results for each category of use are discussed. The categories are organized in order of abundance.

ALIMENTARY PLANTS

For this category of use, 126 citations were recorded for 44 species and 13 different uses (secondary categories).

As expected, the botanical family most represented was Compositae, with 33 citations (26.2% of citations for this category) and 14 species. In order of abundance, these are followed by Liliaceae, with 23 citations (8.3%) and 5 species, Chenopodiaceae, with 15 citations but only one species, Umbelliferae (13 citations, 4 species), and Rosaceae (10 citations, 5 species). Families such as Cruciferae or Labiatae, which are usually very well represented in surveys on alimentary wild plants, had fewer citations.

Table: Alimentary plants – Botanical families

Family	Citations	%	Species
Compositae	33	*26.2*	14
Liliaceae	23	*18.3*	5
Chenopodiaceae	15	*11.9*	1
Umbelliferae	13	*10.3*	4
Rosaceae	10	*7.9*	5
Cruciferae	5	*4.0*	3
Boraginaceae	4	*3.2*	2
Ericaceae	4	*3.2*	1
Others (< 4 citations, 1 species)	19	*15.1*	9

When considering the number of species (21), the alimentary use most cited was, surprisingly, the one that we ourselves defined as a 'rural snack'. This means eating plants as soon as they are gathered, directly in the fields, outside of regular organized meals. This secondary category included plants eaten as fresh fruits or as raw vegetables (tender leaves or stems, the latter sometimes peeled), and also flowers sucked by children in order to savour their sweet sugary nectar. This peculiar way of consuming wild plants has already been pointed out for other Mediterranean countries.

Six species received five or more citations, and most of these were wild relatives of cultivated plants. The species most mentioned was wild asparagus (*Asparagus acutifolius*) with 17 citations and 2 different uses (cooked vegetables, omelettes), followed by wild chard (*Beta vulgaris*) with 15 citations and 2 uses (cooked vegetables, ravioli stuffing), chicory (*Cichorium intybus*) with 8 citations and 3 uses (salads, cooked vegetables, a substitute for coffee), wild fennel (*Foeniculum vulgare* subsp. *piperitum*) with 7 citations and 2 uses (flavouring for canned olives, cooked vegetables), blackberry (*Rubus ulmifolius*) with 5 citations and 3 uses (rural snack, fresh fruits, jam), and *Sonchus tenerrimus* with 5 citations and 3 uses (raw salad, mixed vegetables, rural snack). Most of these plants are commonly used as wild food plants also in many other parts of Italy. Elsewhere, *Sonchus tenerrimus* is more frequently replaced by the more common, close species *Sonchus oleraceus*.

No species was mentioned by all informants. *Asparagus acutifolius* was cited by 12 informants (70.6% of the informants), *Beta vulgaris* was cited by 9 informants (52.9%), and all the remaining species were cited by less than 6 informants. The most frequently used plant parts were leaves from basal rosettes (13 species, 32 citations) and other leaves (6 species, 29 citations), which are eaten mainly as mixed vegetables or raw salads. They were followed by stems (14 species, 19 citations), used as flavouring (*Foeniculum*, *Allium* species), eaten as raw salad, mixed vegetables or rural snack, and fruits (8 species, 18 citations), eaten fresh or dried or are used to prepare jams or a typical syrup (sapa). All the species were easy to find and gather, and mostly grew very close to houses and cultivated fields. Twenty-seven alimentary species (61.4%) were defined by the informants as 'very common'; 13 species (29.5%) as 'moderately common', and only 4 (9.1%) as 'rare'. Most species (32) were found in ruderal anthropic habitats, such as wastelands, marginal areas, courtyards, roadsides. These were followed at a great distance by plants growing in garrigues and shrubs (6 species), wet and shady places (5) and other gathering environments.

According to many of the informants, most alimentary plants are still being gathered by people at the present time.

MEDICINAL PLANTS

In this category, 106 citations were recorded for 40 species and 12 different uses, namely as different general therapeutic indications.

Medicinal plants were found to belong to 23 botanical families. More than one quarter of all citations (24, i.e. 22.6% of all citations) involved Malvaceae, even if only 3 species were mentioned for this family. The next family was Compositae, with 18 citations (17%) and the highest number of species (6, i.e. 15% of medicinal species).

Table: Medicinal plants - Botanical families

Family	Number of citations	*% citations*	Number of species	*% species*
Malvaceae	24	*22,6*	3	*7,5*
Compositae	18	*17,0*	6	*15,0*
Rosaceae	11	*10,4*	5	*12,5*
Liliaceae	8	*7,5*	2	*5,0*
Urticaceae	6	*5,7*	3	*7,5*
Lauraceae	5	*4,7*	1	*2,5*
Oleaceae	5	*4,7*	1	*2,5*
Cactaceae	4	*3,8*	1	*2,5*
others (< 4 citations, 1–2 species)	25	*23,6*	18	*45,0*

The most cited medicinal uses concerned diseases of the digestive system (21 species, 56 citations), followed by injuries (wounds, burns, stings, animals bites, etc.), with 11 species and 16 citations, dermatological affections (9 species, 13 citations), and general state of health (5 species, 13 citations). This last secondary category included plants regarded as effective, not against a specific affection, but in curing and strengthening the body as a whole. Some of these plants are defined as 'cleansing', 'depurant' or 'detoxicant', meaning that they can help in recovering from different diseases by purifying the blood and removing toxins and scum, and possibly by stimulating diuresis. Others are called 'refreshers' or 'anti-inflammables', meaning that they can be effective in relieving pain in the different apparatuses, thanks to their general soothing action and perhaps also by acting as mild laxatives. Such generic and somehow indefinite therapeutic indications are common in ethnobotany, and can be regarded as signs of genuine information.

Malva sylvestris (17 citations, 7 informants) and *Asparagus acutifolius* (7 citations, 7 informants) were found to be the best known and most used medicinal species. Mallow was also found to be the most versatile species (7 different therapeutic indications), while wild asparagus was mentioned only for one use (as a diuretic). *Lavatera cretica* received 6 citations for 6 different uses, but all of them were recorded by only one informant. Indeed, most of the species (27) were mentioned by only one informant, thus revealing that knowledge is unevenly distributed within the community. The most used plant parts are leaves (56 citations, 21 species), followed by flowers and inflorescences (18 citations, 8 species), whole epigeal parts (7, 4), and fruits (4, 4). Note that the prevailing role of leaves is a habitual result in ethnobotanical investigations on medicinal plants carried out in Italy and Europe, while in other parts of the world – for example, in many developing countries – this is not necessarily the case. Remedies are mostly prepared as decoctions (52 citations, 19 species), or used without being prepared (24, 16), prepared as infusions (15, 8) or as poultices (10, 6). Oral dosing, direct application, and giving as food are the most frequently recorded ways of administration. Simplicity in preparing and administering remedies is regarded as a sign of genuine information.

Most of the species were reported by the informants as being 'very common' on Monte Ortobene (24 species, i.e. 60%); 11 species (27.5%) were considered 'moderately common', and only 5 species (12.5%) were termed 'rare'. Almost all the medicinal species (34, i.e. 85%) grow wild in the area; 4 (10%) are cultivated, and 2 (5%) can be found both as wild and as cultivated plants.

Similarly to the alimentary plants reported on, medicinal species are mostly found in ruderal or disturbed habitats (22 species, 55%). Most medicinal plants were reported as having been used in the past, but as not being used any more by the community.

Other Categories

Not many plants and uses were recorded for the remaining categories of use. A short discussion follows.

Domestic

Fifteen species were recorded as being traditionally used in this category, with 23 citations for eight different secondary categories of use. Plants were mainly used for body care, more precisely for rinsing and curing hair. Other uses involved fireplaces and chimneys (twigs used to light a fire or to clean chimneys), scenting rooms or linens, plants used for dyeing clothes or brightening up their colours, repellents for moths or mice, and to make brooms. One informant reported the peculiar use of young shoots of wild olive as a whip to punish children. The most recorded species was *Lavandula stoechas* (4 citations), used both to scent linens and as a repellent against moths.

Ludic

In this category, plants are used – mostly by children – to play games, jokes and as pastimes, or to make toys, dolls and ornaments or fancy-dress costumes. Fifteen species were recorded, with 21 citations for five different secondary categories of use.

Agropastoral

Very few plants and uses were recorded for this category (7 species, 8 citations, 5 uses). *Opuntia* branches are planted to serve as fences; cut-off branches of other thorny plants are placed above typical dry-stone walls (*sa cresura*) to keep people and/or animals out. Plants are also used in sheep farming, pork butchering, wine producing, and to make certain agricultural tools.

Magical/Medicinal

For this category, six citations were recorded, for five species and two different uses. While the magical use of plants to heal warts is frequent in many parts of Italy, the rite for treating jaundice reported by one informant is very peculiar. Jaundice is known locally as *su male 'e s'istria* (which means 'barn owl's disease'), because the coming of a barn owl is believed to portend this illness. Four different plants (*Artemisia arborescens*, *Helychrysum italicum* and blessed olive and palm tree leaves), together with salt and holy water, are involved in this complicated rite, which must be performed by a healer and repeated for three days.

Indeed, it should also be noted that the use of many medicinal plants also includes some magical aspects in collecting the plants and/or in preparing and administering the remedies.

Religious

Seven citations were recorded for this category. Four plants were reported as being used to decorate altars on various feast days (Christmas, Easter, Corpus Christi).

Handicrafts

Only two citations for two ethnobotanical uses (stools and baskets) were mentioned by the informants for this category.

Magical/ritual/propitiatory

Two traditional magical uses of plants were recorded: a propitiatory agricultural practice to keep birds away from sown fields, and predictions regarding future husbands for young women.

Further Information

During the investigation, further information was also collected. It is reported here in a separate section, either because the data are incomplete, or because they are not of strictly ethnobotanical interest (e. g. traditional cookies prepared with almonds, which come from cultivated trees and are normally used in this way).

Ornamental Plants

A few informants reported the usage of picking up wild flowers to decorate houses. The following species were mentioned:

- *Cyclamen repandum* S. et S.
- *Dactylorhiza insularis* (Sommier) Landwehr
- *Lupinus angustifolius* L.
- *Ophrys incubacea* Bianca
- *Orchis longicornu* Poiret
- *Orchis papilionacea* L.
- *Petrorhagia velutina* (Guss) P.W. Ball & Heywood
- *Ranunculus* cfr. *monspeliacus* L.

In fact, it is very likely that many other plants are commonly collected for this purpose – perhaps all those with colored or attractive flowers – and possibly even the same informants would have mentioned different species if they had been interviewed in a different season.

TOXIC PLANTS

The following plants were pointed out as being poisonous or potentially toxic for humans or livestock:

- *Arbutus unedo* L. (eating too many fruits may cause nausea and vomiting)
- *Asparagus acutifolius* L. (people suffering from diabetes, hypertension or renal troubles are advised not to eat too many sprouts by way of vegetables)
- *Ferula communis* L. (this plant is poisonous for sheep)
- *Papaver rhoeas* L. (the excessive use of seeds as a soporific for babies may cause convulsions)

TRADITIONAL BISCUITS

Some biscuits traditionally prepared with almonds for special festivities were reported by a few informants, together with recipes and related customs.

One of these customs (see: *papassinos*) is particularly interesting, as it is very similar to the traditional American celebration of Halloween.

Guerfos

Prepared with sweet and bitter almonds (finely chopped), sugar, honey, lemon peel and some brandy. All the ingredients are combined together and cooked until the mixture is thick enough to make small, compact spheres that will be sprinkled with icing sugar. The same mixture is used to stuff a candied citrus fruit called *pompia. Guerfos*, which are typically made for baptisms and weddings, are nowadays prepared and consumed for no special occasion, but throughout the year. For traditional weddings, the bridegroom used to bring to the bride's house 12 hearts made of pastry stuffed with the *guerfos* mixture.

Zarminu

Similar to meringues, these cookies are prepared with egg whites beaten with sugar. The batter is shaped into small rounds with toasted and sliced almonds at the centre of each round, then put in the oven to bake. Before serving, the *zarminu* are trimmed with small silver-colored ornaments called *trazzea.* They are typically made for parties and receptions.

Papassinos

Prepared with water, wheat flour, lard, almonds, walnuts and raisins, mixed together. The pastry is rolled and cut into small rhombs that are baked in the oven, then iced with a mixture of egg whites and sugar, and lastly trimmed with colored *trazzea.*

These are made typically for All Souls' Day (November 2nd). The evening before All Souls, children visit the neighbouring houses knocking on doors and ask, '*Su mortu, mortu*?' (i.e. 'Is the dead dead?'). In the past, housewives replied to this request by giving almonds, walnuts, dried figs, pomegranates, quinces or *papassinos* to the children; nowadays, the fruits and sweets have been replaced by coins.

Sa Arantzada

Prepared with orange peel, boiled, cut into small strips and mixed with heated honey and almonds. This mixture is also used to stuff the candied citrus called *pompia.* Typically prepared for baptism parties.

Amarettos

Sweet almonds are chopped, and are then mixed with egg whites, flour, sugar and a few bitter almonds. The pastry is shaped into round biscuits, which are then baked in the oven. Prepared for weddings, baptisms and important festivities.

Sayings

Allium triquetrum (in local language: apara).

There is a traditional joking metaphor: 'S'este falau chie s'apara' (i. e.: 'It wilted like wild garlic'), referring to 'something' that, after 'blooming', looses all vigour and appeal. In fact, the inflorescence of this plant quickly wilts in the presence of heat or when picked.

Reichardia picroides (in local language: mammalucca).

The words *mammalucca* (for women) and *mammaluccu* (for men) are also used to designate stupid people.

CONCLUSION

The information collected at Monte Ortobene and presented here shows that a certain richness and diversity of knowledge regarding traditional uses for plants still survives as a part of the cultural heritage of the community. However, this knowledge is ageing, and is likely to vanish fairly soon. As reported by most of the informants, many practices are no longer in use and survive only as memories from the past. Even on the basis of a small number of informants, this pattern is particularly clear in medicinal uses (see, for instance, the large number of plants cited by fewer than 3 informants), and is confirmed by the results of the quantitative analyses. It is clear that these traditional phytotherapeutic remedies were more popular and widespread in the past, when medicines were not easily available. At present it is not surprising that, for the sake of their own health, people have a greater faith in 'official' medicines prescribed by doctors than they do in folk remedies. On the contrary, several edible wild plants are still gathered and processed by members of the community, and many of these plants are popular both as delicacies and as the ingredients of local specialties.

In general, in the Monte Ortobene area as in other Mediterranean zones, the younger generations have lost much of the traditional knowledge necessary for identifying, gathering and treating wild plant species. It is thus becoming crucial that this biocultural diversity be recorded and preserved by means of proper documentation and an identification of the relative species before it vanishes definitively. It is also of great importance to consider this cultural heritage within the framework of a sustainable management approach, with the aim of preserving all the components of its environmental diversity.

12

Ethnobotany in the Nepal Himalaya

BACKGROUND

The term ethnobotany was coined by John W. Harsberger in 1896 and was considered as the art of collection of useful plants by a group of people and the description of the uses of plants. Ford developed the science of ethnobotanical study and included the understanding of knowledge systems through the use of anthropological methods. Over the last century, ethnobotany has evolved into a scientific discipline that focuses on the people-plant relationship in a multidisciplinary manner, incorporating not only collection and documentation of indigenous uses but also ecology, economy, pharmacology, public health, and other disciplines. Presently, ethnobotany has become increasingly valuable in the development of health care and conservation programs in different parts of the world. Ethnobotanical studies that explore and help to preserve knowledge are therefore urgently needed before traditional folklores are lost ever.

Ethnomedicine, a branch of ethnobotany, is a set of empirical local practices embedded in the indigenous knowledge of a social group often transmitted orally from generation to generation with intent to understand social, cultural, and economic factors influencing health problems and to overcome such problems. It is a suitable source of information regarding useful medicinal plants that can be targeted for sustainable domestication and management. Ethnobotany and ethnomedicine as sciences addressing indigenous knowledge and practices therefore are now very important for establishing management programs.

Justification

The dialectical relationship between indigenous knowledge and practices shape, the ecosystem and affects the constituent plant populations. By incorporating indigenous knowledge and use in the process of scientific research, new hypotheses for the sustainable conservation of the resources can be developed. Indigenous knowledge and use have to be analyzed to develop appropriate management measures that build on both scientific and local knowledge. Due to changing perception of the local people, and the ever increasing influence of global commercialization and socio-economic transformation, indigenous knowledge on plant resource use is constantly diminishing. Due to the lack of organized sustainable and scientifically monitored cultivation and harvesting, proper management techniques, and lack of awareness of social factors, the number of useful plant resources is decreasing at an alarming rate. Furthermore, the indigenous knowledge on the use of lesser-known plants is also rapidly declining. The present study therefore reviews the indigenous knowledge and use of plant resources of Nepal Himalayas along the altitudinal and longitudinal gradient, an area so far unstudied in Nepal.

Context

The first scientific study of Nepalese useful and medicinal plants was conducted by Francis Buchanan, who collected plants from 1802–1803. He was followed by Nathaniel Wallich 1820–1821. Don and Wallich also collected plants in the Nepal Himalayas and recorded their uses. The earliest published ethnomedicinal-botanical study of Nepal was a paper on medicinal and food plants from eastern Nepal by Banerji. His study was followed by many other researches. Since the 1980s, extensive ethnobotanical studies were conducted. However, none of them has analyzed patterns of the usage of plant resources along the altitudinal and longitudinal gradient. All previous studies enumerated only the plant diversity and usage of plant resources of selected small sites and selected tribal groups, without attempting to synthesize the plant use information in Nepal.

REVIEW AND FIELD VISITS

A total of 264 studies, with emphasis on ethnobotany, ethnomedicine, and diversity of medicinal and aromatic plants, conducted between 1979 to 2006, were consulted for the present analysis. Of these papers only 76 were including data on the diversity and distribution of medicinal and aromatic plants, ethnobotany, as well as aspects of ethnomedicine and conservation. Four field visits were carried out in May and December 2006, January--February 2007 and April–May 2008, focusing on the Baglung, Baitadi, Dadeldhura, Darchula, Doti, Gulmi, and Kanchanpur districts of west Nepal, stretching from 80°5' to 83°15' E longitude 28°27' 30" to 30°15' N latitude and 390 m to 4570 m altitude. Field visits were meant for data verification and cross checking.

Nepal extends along the Himalayan range between the latitudes 26°22' – 30°27' and longitudes 80°04' – 88°12'. Altitudes vary from less than 60 m in the lowland of Terai in the South to the crest of the Himalaya reaching 8848 m in the North. In the present study, for easier interpretation and analysis along the longitudinal gradient, the country's longitude was divided into three bio-geographical regions: West Nepal (80°E to 83°E), Central Nepal (83°E to 86°E) and East Nepal (86°E to 88°E). An analysis of the altitudinal gradient was made in 1000 m intervals as 60 – 1000 m, 1000 – 2000 m, 2000 – 3000 m, and 3000 – 4000 m.

RESULTS AND DISCUSSION

History and Plant Usage

Plants have been one of the most important sources of food and medicine since the dawn of human civilization. Archaeological evidence of 60,000 year-old Neanderthal burial grounds in Shanidar,

Iraq, points to the use of plants like Marshmallow, Yarrow and Groundsel, which are still used in contemporary folk medicine. Evidence for the medicinal use of *Papaver somniferum*, the opium poppy, dates back 8000 years. Concomitantly, the earliest written record of plants used as medicine originating from the Himalayas are found in the 6,500 year old texts of the Rigveda, followed by Atharveveda (2000-1000 BC) and Auryveda (600-100 BC). The oldest account recording the uses of 278 Nepalese medicinal plants is 'Saushrut Nighantu,' written in 878 AD (935 BS). Later 'Nepali Nighantu,' an elaborated encyclopedia with information on the traditional knowledge of 750 plant species was published by the Royal Nepal Academy in 1969.

Until the middle of the 19th century, plants were the main therapeutic agents used by humans, and even today almost 80% of the world population rely to some extent on medicinal plants for their primary healthcare needs. The use of nearly 3000 plant species as food during the course of human civilization has been documented, but only about 150 species have been cultivated and less that 10 plant species are meeting over 90% of the world food demand. Human survival still can not be imagined without plants. The importance of plants is substantial and reflected in the large variety of products such as food, fiber, fodder, vegetables, medicinal plants, and aromatic plants. The contribution of medicinal plants in Nepal is important. A total of 1012 useful plants are documented for Nepal, of which 554 (54.74%) have ethnomedicinal in properties. An review of research conducted in the Nepal Himalayas indicated that nearly 40% of the studies were related to medicinal plants and ethnomedicine, underlining that ethnomedicine is utmost important in the Nepal Himalayas.

MEDICINAL PLANTS AND THEIR DISTRIBUTION

About 60% of the world population and 60–90% of the population of developing countries (80% in Nepal, 70% in India, 80% in Pakistan, 65% in Sri Lanka, 90% in Bangladesh, 85% in Burma, and 60% in Indonesia rely on traditional medicine, and about 85% of the traditional remedies for primary health care are derived from plants.

In the world, 10–18% of all plant species are used medicinally while in Nepal medicinal plants account about 20–28% of the local flora. The data for India and China is significantly higher i.e. 44% and 29–41% respectively. The present analysis found that an average of 56% of higher plants were ethnobotanically important, and 54% were used as ethnomedicine in the Nepal Himalayas. This indicates that there are more ethnobotanically and ethnomedicinally important plant species in the Nepal Himalayas than previously estimated. Similar accounts of a much higher incidence of plants used in ethnomedicine (more than the estimated 10–18% was recorded all over the world; e.g. about 24% in Costa Rica, 25–42% in Kenya, 27% in Israel, 31–51% in Brazil, and 46% in Guyana, 64% in Jammu Kashmir, India, 54% in Similipahar, Orissa, India, and 48% in Beni, Bolivia.

Table: Ethnobotanical and ethnomedicinal plants in the world

SN	Location and total no. of higher plants	Ethnobotanical plants as % of total flora	Ethnomedicinal plants
1	Nepal, 7000	28%	21% of total flowering plants
2	Nepal, 7000	56.35% *	53.59% of total plants in use
3	Hindu Kush Himalaya, 25000	33–40%	
4	Indian Himalaya, 8000		21% of total flowering plants
5	India, 17000	14%	44% of total flowering plants
6	Pakistan, 6000		12% of total flowering plants
7	China, 29700		41% of total flowering plants
8	World, 297000 <		10–18% of total plants

* Percentage of plants used in terms of species richness of sites

Asia represents one of the most important centers of knowledge with regard to the use of plant species for treatment of various diseases. Examples are the Ayurveda, Amchi (traditional healing system of Tibet and mountain areas of Nepal), Siddha, Unani, and Chinese systems of medical care. Folklore medicinal systems (traditional healing and faith healing) are also important in Nepal. In this context, it is interesting to note that the Himalayan medicinal plants are the major contributors to the aforementioned systems. The topographical characteristics of the Himalayas have resulted in a variety of ecological niches that host diverse medicinal plants. It has been estimated that the Himalayan region harbors over 10,000 species of medicinal and aromatic plants, supporting the livelihoods of about 600 million people living in the area. The Nepal Himalayas include about 2,000 species with medicinal and aromatic values, and more than 1,400 of these are known to be used locally particularly as medicines.

Medicinal and aromatic plant species richness increases along increasing altitude up to 2000 m and then continues to decline. The temperate and alpine zones harbor highly valued medicinal plants. The diversity of medicinal plants in a mid elevation peak model, was comparable to other studies. Bhattarai and Vetaas highlighted an insignificant relationship between herbaceous species richness and elevation and climatic factors in the Himalayas.

The distribution of medicinal herbs at high altitudes is mainly controlled by both environmental and ecophysiological factors. The maximum species richness at 1000–2000 m could be associated with optimum energy and rainfall. The hard boundary effect might also influence the species richness at high elevation. The trans-Himalaya ecosystem is a fragile biome, characterized by a reduced growing season, low productivity, high intensity of solar radiation, and high degree of resource seasonality, resulting in the control of distribution, richness, physiological stress, and metabolic compounds of medicinal plants. The high altitude medicinal plants contain secondary metabolic compounds as an adaptive strategy to reduce the damaging effects.

ETHNOBOTANY AND ETHNOMEDICINE

Many people use plants as remedies as an alternative or in addition to visiting western health care practitioners. The extent of plant use differs with location. The use of plants for subsistence, medicines, and source for supplementary income is highly variable. About 85% of the rural population of Nepal are said to use herbal remedies. The use of plant resources as herbal remedies is especially important at higher altitudes. We found that the percentage of plants used as medicine increased along increasing altitude but there was no significant trend in increased usage of plants for other purposes. The overall plant use was proportionate to the number of plant species used in ethnomedicine.

A positive correlation between species richness and number of ethnobotanically useful plants was found, but the relationship was not significant. In contrast, a significant positive correlation was found by Salick et al. The ethnobotanical use as percentage of plant species richness (number of enumerated plant species) decreased from east to west Nepal, whereas the ethnomedicinal usage increased from east to west Nepal. Though there was a record of the lowest number of medicinal plants in west Nepal, we found the highest usage of plants as ethnomedicine from the same region. Similar relationships were found by other studies. The reason for this could be the excessive utilization of local plant resources as remedies. Lack of modern facilities and services and less development in west Nepal compel the population to use existing plant resources for their immediate needs. Eastern Nepal is comparatively moister than western Nepal and the moisture gradient accounts for differences in plant species richness.

High altitude medicinal plants provide quality products, and this is the reason why they are often the first choice of local users as immediate therapy and by pharmaceutical companies as precious ingredients. Our analysis shows that the proportion of usage of plants as ethnomedicine steadily increased with increasing altitude. Pohlefound, however, an insignificant relationship between the diversity of the flora and the number of wild plants used by local people in mid hills. Higher uses of plants as ethnomedicine at higher altitude was attributed to the absence of modern medical facilities, and intensive uses of plants as remedies in mountain areas. In remote and high altitude areas, medicinal herbs are the main ingredients of local medicines and the traditional health care system is considered as the main lifeline and frequently the first choice. There is greater dependence among the population upon natural resources. The optimum uses of the limited plant resources revealed a higher percentage of uses in high altitude areas.

However, this trend could not be observed in lowland Terai. The usage of plants as ethnomedicine was less in Terai, with the richness of flowering plants and medicinal plant was higher. The low number (48.96%) of ethnomedicinal plants found in Terai was consistent with the findings of Bishokarma et al (35.15%) from the same site. Lesser usage of local plants for therapy was attributed to the availability and accessibility of infrastructures, communication, transport, development, and as such less dependant on the availability of plant resources; but a higher preferences towards allopathic medicines. It was also associated with limited knowledge and limited skilled individuals. However, some marginalized communities and tribal groups of lowland Terai, with poor access to the modern medical facilities, were still utilizing local plant resources for local therapy. Subsequently, most communities still use folk herbal remedies as a readily and cheaply available alternative. A decline of the traditional knowledge has been underway for hundreds of years, and the knowledge on medicinal plant use is clearly disappearing fast in low lands of Nepal.

The higher percentage of ethnomedicinal uses of plants in high altitude areas was due to the preferences given by local people to the traditional herbal remedies, and a situation of having no alternative choices, as well as poverty and belief in the effectiveness of folklore herbal remedies. The greater usage of plants as herbal remedies in mountain areas is also due to the prevalence of traditional health systems such as folklore medicinal systems and the Amchi system. The traditional healing systems are both culturally acceptable and induce locales to use plant resource most. Because of the high level of cohesion and strong cultural links with nature in mountain areas, local people have a close affinity with locally available resources and easily internalize the resources for their livelihood and needs because these are also readily available.

Home herbal treatment is not merely a medical system but a part of culture, and the extensive use of locally available plant resources was observed in mountain areas. Most of the people of mountain areas, particularly elderly people, farmers, and mid-wives, are well acquainted to medicinal herbs and their usage, and plants are prescribed to the patients whenever required. The availability of traditional healers is also higher in rural and mountain areas. The use of herbal remedies in mountain areas to alleviate suffering is perhaps as old as the origin of man itself, and there is a general trend of increase in the use of medicinal plants.

Besides health care and subsistence uses, medicinal plants have a high potential as alternative income-generating sources of the rural hilly populace of the region. Therefore, sustainable use of the resources and conservation of indigenous knowledge of medicinal plants may compliment the income of local people. Medicinal plants are mainly harvested in the wild, traded, and eventually consumed as processed form in lowland cities. Up to 50% of the Nepal's rural household's income is derived from commercial collection of medicinal and aromatic plants. The collection of medicinal plants in a sustainable manner is an integrated process with potential for development and conservation.

The indigenous knowledge and practice of usage of medicinal plants in rural areas of Nepal is passed down through oral tradition and personal experiences. The knowledge clearly decreased with age. People of ages between 40–60 possessed greater knowledge on identification and uses of medicinal and aromatic plants in Nepal Himalaya, which was consistent to the observation of Philips and Gentry. The young generations tend to leave ancestral practices behind, refocusing their interests on treatments offered by western medicine. Due to changing lifestyles, perception as well as social transformation, the plant resource and indigenous knowledge of utilization are being severely degraded. This impact is inevitable to the Nepal Himalayas and plant resources are in great peril. Indigenous knowledge systems are not only of value for the cultures from which they evolve, but also for scientists and planners striving to improve the living conditions in rural societies. Lambert et al pointed out that preserving and enhancing the indigenous plant knowledge and use was equivalent to 'rescuing a global heritage'. Indigenous plant based traditional knowledge and use has become a recognized tool in search for new sources of drugs and pharmaceuticals. In countries like Kenya and Nepal, where the indigenous knowledge is predominantly used for utilization of plant resource for various purposes, and high priority needs to be given to the documentation of indigenous knowledge and use of plant resources to help their conservation.

CONCLUSION

The richness of medicinal plants was decreasing with increasing altitude, but the percentage of plants used as medicine steadily increased with increasing altitude. This was due to preferences given to herbal remedies in high altitude areas and a situation of having no alternative choices, poverty and belief on effectiveness of folklore herbal remedies. Enhancing the sustainable use and conservation of indigenous knowledge of useful and medicinal plants may benefit and improve the living standard of poor people.

13

Living Knowledge of the Healing Plants

Contribution of indigenous knowledge in developing more effective drugs with minimum or no side effects helped to realise importance of study of indigenous remedies and the conservation of biological resources. This study analysed indigenous knowledge regarding medicinal plants use among the Chepang communities from ward number 3 and 4 of Shaktikhor Village Development Committee located in the central mid hills of Nepal.

Data were collected in a one-year period and included interviews with traditional healers and elders. Chepangs are rich in knowledge regarding use of different plants and were using a total 219 plant parts from 115 species including one mushroom (belonging 55 families) for medicinal uses.

Out of these, 75 species had 118 different new medicinal uses and 18 of them were not reported in any previous documents from Nepal as medicinal plants.

Spiritual belief, economy and limitation of alternative health facilities were cause of continuity of people's dependency on traditional healers. Change in socio-economic activities not only threatened traditional knowledge but also resource base of the area. Enforcement of local institution in management of forest resources and legitimating traditional knowledge and practices could help to preserve indigenous knowledge.

BACKGROUND

The close and traditional dependence of many indigenous and local communities on biological resources and its importance in conservation and development is now being recognised widely. The growing appreciation of the value of traditional knowledge is due to its importance to development, conservation and other wide range of uses also for other people than those who are traditionally dependent on it. Traditional knowledge that built upon the long experiences of people was adopted in social, economic, environmental, spiritual and political practices. Since traditional knowledge is developed through a long trail and error, this could guide search for new drugs. Together with the recognition of importance of traditional knowledge, serious concern about the loss of knowledge could be observed in last few years throughout the world. Chepangs lived a semi-nomadic life, more dependent on the forests. They have generated enormous knowledge on a large number of plants species on which they have depended for centuries. Due to this, forests were most important resources for them in terms of food, fibre, medicine, housing materials, fodder and various other needs. The loss of knowledge could also threat the existing balance between these people and natural environment.

Despite many studies on various uses of plants a large number of plants and associated traditional uses still wait proper documentation. This is perhaps because of the fact that these studies do not fully represent the wide range of environments in Nepal, where topography has created diverse ecological niches for species and stirred localized cultural constructions. In Chepang areas also documentation of ethonobotanical knowledge was limited to a few medicinal plants. This study helped to document knowledge of several medicinal herbs use including many new reports for Nepal.

CHEPANGS

There are approximately 52,000 Chepangs in 2000 and their habitats are quite identical and found along the Trisuli, Narayani and

Rapti Rivers and in the major catchments of their tributaries covering the adjoining frontiers of Dhading, Makwanpur, Chitwan and Gorkha districts of central Nepal. Being hunter-gatherers until about 80 years ago, the Chepang are considered among the most primitive indigenous peoples of Nepal. They practise shifting cultivation (Slash and burn cultivation) and the evidence suggests that they are highly forest-dependent as well as among the poorest in Nepal and besides their own use of forest resources such as timber, herbs and wild food, they barter and some times sell forest products. The forest is used as an important source of food, fibre, medicine, housing materials, fuel and fodder. They are generally considered to be shy and easily dominated by other ethnic groups, who have been migrating from the mountains to the lowlands for the last 40–50 years.

METHODOLOGY

Study Area

This study was conducted in two villages in ward no. 3 and 4 of Shaktikhor Village Development Committee (VDC) (27°40'E-27°48'E and 84°35'N-84°39'N) of Chitwan District in the Central Nepal. Though these two areas belong to the same VDC, they are in different climatic zone and have different situation of access. The population distribution is also not homogeneous but dependency on forest is common in both areas. The distribution of Chepangs is similar in these two areas. The ward number 3 is accessible from road whereas ward number 4 is on the top of the hill at one day long walking distance with no road access. The Climatic zone includes Tropical to subtropical. The altitude of this village varies from 300 m to 2500 m asl. The vegetation of this area includes lowland Sal forest, hill Sal forest, *Schima wallichi* forest, tropical riverine forest, tropical mixed broadleaved forest and subtropical mixed forest.

Methods

Study took place between 1 June 2001 and 31 May 2002. Basically, semi-structured interviews were conducted with key informants like traditional healers for medicinal plants, and elder people and women for edible and other useful plants. Initial rapport-building visits included discussions with local leaders, traditional healers and other key informants as well as community-wide meetings introducing the research activity and its purpose. This helped to identify key informants (2 traditional healers both man and 10 elders of which 4 female and 6 male all above 60 years old). The 'artefact/interview' approach was also used, i.e. asking questions about the use of plants for different purposes and making forest visits to identify the plant species. During forest visits, queries were made on plants not mentioned in the interviews, to trap the knowledge of forgotten species. Since Chepangs are very shy, a trained local assistant was used to facilitate the interviews. In interview, information on use of various medicinal plants to cure different illness, plant part used, use methods and their faith on traditional healers were acquired. Interview was mainly in Nepali but when they find difficulties to explain or understand any thing then the local assistant helped to interpret. Few old Chepangs were not confident of Nepali language so interpreter helped to interpret question as well as answer. Preparation method of any medicinal herb varies for different illness and also seriousness of the illness. Moreover, traditional faith healers were reluctant to explain mode of preparation of herbs for serious illnesses to avoid potential casualties from inexperienced person. Therefore, mode of preparation is not included in this report.

Plant parts having multiple use are counted for each use. Supply column in the indicates source of supply (i.e. from wild or from the garden). Author identified plants using his more than 20 years experience from botanical studies in different parts of Nepal. Herbarium specimens were prepared following standard botanical procedure for only new specimens or specimen that needed further confirmation. The confusing species were confirmed by tallying with the herbarium at the National Herbarium and Plant Research Department (Kath), Godawari, Nepal. Plant names follows Press et al. 2000. Secondary information involves publication on information of the study area, ethnobotanical studies of Chepangs, and medicinal plants studies in Nepal. To confirm new reports for Nepal, findings were compared with all published information from Nepal including bulletins of Department of Medicinal plants of Nepal. A name list of permanent residents of ward no. 3 and 4 that was made available by Village Development Committee (VDC) was used to group them into sex and five age classes (< 20, 21–30, 31–40, 41–50, > 50 yrs) for each ward. From this list, 12 individuals were drawn randomly from each age class of both sex for each ward ($n = 2 \times 5 \times 12 \times 2 = 240$) and interviewed for their knowledge of medicinal plant use. Total Chepang population in these two wards was 168 household i.e. 1008 individuals. The sample size represent 24% of the total Cheapang population. The knowledge difference between youth and elder people and the transmission of knowledge was analysed through mixed linear regression analysis at 95% confidence interval of knowledge for each age class, sex and ward.

The use of 95% confidence interval is justified by there being a tradition that all age groups are involved in plant use and good sharing of knowledge. For several causes affecting knowledge, justifications were obtained from elder Chepangs and relevant secondary sources. Estimates from the statistical analysis of plant use knowledge for each sex of all age groups from both wards were plotted against the age groups to explain graphically the knowledge distribution among each sex from both wards for all age groups. Similarly, average plant use knowledge for each uses was calculated to see knowledge difference in each uses. Standard deviation of each uses for each sex was also calculated to analyse magnitude of differences within each sex of both wards.

Table: Average medicinal plant use knowledge among male and female of ward number 3 & 4 of Shaktikhor VDC.

Ward	Sex	Medicine
3	M	130.9 ± (64.7)
3	F	96.6 ± (63.6)
4	M	111 ± (59.1)
4	F	117.2 ± (66.6)

The values in the parenthesis are standard deviation.

Table: Models describing variation in plant use knowledge.

Model describing the variation of medicinal plant use knowledge among different age groups, sex and wards (LS Means). **N = 240, σ^2 = 493.81, σ = 22.22, df = 106**			
Effect	**Estimate**	**Standard Error**	**Pr > |t|**
Intercept	185.6	48.21	< 0.0002
Age	6.9479	0.3765	< 0.0001
Sex F	105.75	2.7610	0.0001
Sex M	122.08	2.7611	0.0001
Ward 3	113.66	2.7615	0.0001
Ward 4	114.17	2.7606	0.0001
Sex F*Ward 3	-37.55	9.259	0.0001
Sex M*Ward 3	0	.	.
Sex F*Ward 4	0	.	.
Sex M*Ward 4	0	.	.

RESULTS

Plant Use

A total 219 plant parts from 115 species (belonging 55 families) including one mushroom were in use among Chepang for medicinal uses. Of them 29 are trees, 36 shrubs, 25 herbs, 21 climbers, 3 ferns and one fungi (mushroom). These belong to 105 genera and 55 families.

Of the plants in use among Chepangs, 75 species had 118 different new medicinal uses for Nepal and 18 of them were not reported in any previous documents from Nepal as medicinal plants. Number of plant used to treat fever was highest (17 species) followed by wound, diarrhoea and indigestion (14 to each). Of these 115 species, 107 are wild, 7 cultivated and 1 both wild as well as cultivated. Responding question regarding faith on traditional healers, all respondent (except few youth) expressed their faith.

Plant parts use indicated that the root/thizome had the highest use (45) followed by bark (39), fruit (32) and leaf (32). In some plants more than one part are used to cure various illnesses. Of these, 7 species were found cultivated, 107 species were collected from the wild and 1 species was found both in wild as well as planted. Detail results with species name, local name, part(s) used, ailments treated are tabulated.

To maintain regeneration, traditional harvest practice was found leaving some flowers for seed formation, whole aerial part collection of annuals only after dispersal of seed and leaving some roots or tubers or bulbs for regeneration.

Table: Plant parts use.

Plant part	No. of uses
Bark	38
Root/rhizome	45
Tuber/bulb	10
Flower/inflorescence	2
Fruit	32
Seed/Grain	9
Oil/Butter	1
Latex/sap	11
Leaf	33
Stem/Stem fibre	17
Tender shoot	20
Whole plant	1
Total parts used	219

Of the 115 medicinal use species, 9 belong to different IUCN threat categories. These falls within four threat categories and altogether 13 different parts of these species were in use among Chepang communities. Of the 9 threatened species, 4 are tree, 2 shrub, 2 climber and 1 herb.

Species use and plant part use indicated that there were many species for common illnesses like Indigestion (18 species), Fever (17 species) and wound (15 species).

Table: Threatened species in use.

Species	Habit	IUCN Threat category	Plant Part Used	Medicinal uses	Other uses*	Total number of uses
Acacia catechu (L.f.) Willd.	Tree	CT	Stem, bark	2	2	4
Alstonia scholaris (L.) R.Br.	Tree	R	Latex, stem	1	1	2
Bergenia ciliata (Haw.) Stemb.	Herb	CT	Rhizome	4	1	5
Crateva unilocularis Buch.-Ham.	Tree	R	Bark, shoot	1	2	3
Dioscorea deltoidea Wall. Ex Griseb	Climber	CT	Tuber	1	2	3
Dioscorea prazeri Prain & Burkill	Climber	CT	Tuber	1	2	3
Oroxylum indicum (L.) Kurz.	Tree	V	Seed	1	0	1
Rauvolfia serpentina (L.) Benth. ex Kurz	Shrub	E	Root, leaf	2	1	3
Swertia chirayita (Roxb.ex Fleming) H. Karst.	Shrub	V	Whole plant	1	1	2

*Other uses include uses other than medicinal (source: Rijal, 2007).

CT = Commercially Threatened, R = Rare, V = Vulnerable, E = Endangered.

Table: Number of plants for each illness.

Illness	Plant parts in used	Number of plant used
Abdominal spasm	9	9
Abortion	1	1
Antihelmintic	13	13
Asthama	2	2
Body ache	2	2
Boils	1	1
Burn	4	4
Chest pain	3	3
Cholera	2	2
Cold	8	8
Constipation	3	3
Cough	11	11
Cuts	2	2
Dealcoholisation	1	1
Diarrhoea	15	12
Dysentery	13	13
Enuresis	1	1
Fever	17	17
Fracture	7	6
Gastric	1	1
Heart pain	1	1
Heat sickness	11	11
Herpes zoster	1	1
Indigestion	18	18
Inflamation	1	1
Insecticide	4	4
Internal heat sickness	1	1
Liver problem	1	1
Loss of weight	3	3
Malaria	1	1

Malnourishment	2	2
Menopause	1	1
Miscariage	1	1
Oedema	1	1
Pneumonia	2	2
Psynocytis	3	3
Snake bite	5	5
Sprain	2	2
Scabies	1	1
Scorpion sting	2	2
Stomachic	6	6
Taenia pedis	2	2
Teeth infection	4	4
Throat problem	1	1
Tonic	6	6
Typhoid	3	3
Urine infection	2	2
Vomiting	2	2
Wound	15	15
Total	219	215*

*Since several species have multiple uses, total count counted species more than once (for each remedy) and due to that total became 215 which in reality is only 115 species.

KNOWLEDGE DISTRIBUTION

Model of all ages of both sexes from two wards:

$$Y_i = ì_0 + á.age_j + â.sex_k + ã.sex_k(ward_l) + å_i$$

Where i = 1......240; j = 1......54, k = 1, 2, l = 1, 2, Y = medicinal plant use knowledge (number); $ì_0$, $á_{age(j)}$, $â_{sex(k)}$ and $ã_{sexl(wardk)}$ are model parameters and $å_i$ is the residual term ($å_i$~N (0,$ó^2$)).

Statistical analysis model indicated that age, sex and interaction of sex and ward has significant effect on knowledge regarding medicinal plants.

DISCUSSION

Herbal Knowledge

Compare to other ethnic groups of Nepal, Chepangs of Shaktikhor were found very knowledgeable in use of plant for various need of livelihood. This indicates close affinity of these people with plants of the area. The number of plant in use (115 species) was found higher compared to the reports from different ethnic groups of Nepal except the Tharu communities of Chitwan District. From the use diversity aspects, it is highest (219) then earlier highest use (185) among Tharus of Chitwan [ibid.]. Although Khan, 1998 also studied these communities, he was able to report only 19 medicinal plants in use but realised limitation of his study (only one day fieldwork) and suggested for more in-depth study. No new medicinal use for Nepal was reported in earlier studies of Chepangs. Therefore, this study has contributed to bring more information on traditional medicinal plant use knowledge with the record of 120 new medicinal uses of 75 different species of which 18 species were not reported in any previous documents from Nepal as medicinal plants.

Dependency

Like in many other rural communities, their faith was reason for continuing herbal treatment. Chepangs belief that holy spirits live in plants, animals, rivers and mountains. According to their beliefs, disease and natural disasters are caused by disrespect of the spirits. Due to such belief they have faith on *Pande* or *Phal* or *Janne* (traditional faith healers) and for preference to go to them to treat illness through spiritual practices. Besides, accessibility and economic reasons had also forced them to depend on traditional healing practice. The health post with only health assistant was established in this area very recently and is far from the village. The health post receives very limited medicine from the government and mainly for common diseases or wounds. Since most of the Chepangs were familiar with herbs of common remedies (fever, cough, cold, headache, stomach ache, body pain, heat sickness, constipation, internal heat sensation, weakness, indigestion, sprain, anti-helmintic, scabies, psynocytis, herpes zoster, burn, teeth infection, vomiting and dealcoholisation, minor diarrhoea/dysentery) they rather prefer to use herbs then visiting health post.

In some serious cases of the illness like diarrhoea/dysentery, sprain, psynocysis, burn or vomiting, and other special cases like snake bite, scorpion sting, fracture, pneumonia, liver/heart/lung/ kidney problems, typhoid, taenia pedis, malnourishment, urine or other infection, malaria, abortion, inflammation, miscarriage and cholera they visit traditional faith healer *(Pande/Pha//Janne).* The plant parts and species use also indicated high number of species and plant parts use for remedy of common illnesses. They visit health posts only if the *Pande/Pha//Janne* advice in serious cases but they usually don't get much help as health post doesn't have doctor but only health assistant. As mentioned by Gurung, 1995, villagers of this area also informed that there had been several cases in which people returned to the traditional healers when illness was not cured by modern medicine. The limited medical services in health post, poor economy and belief in faith on traditional healers are the cause of returning to traditional healers. Moreover, traditional practice was cheaper as payment could be made with goods like chicken or/and food grains which are available at their home.

CONSERVATION AND PLANT USE

The plant part use examination showed that root/rhizome is used in a large number of species followed by bark use. Root/ rhizome and stem collection if not done carefully then could threaten existence of the species. Debarking or collection of sap/latex could threat the tree if practiced inappropriately. Even more sensitive is the collection of root, rhizome, tuber and bulb. It is learned from the local residents that a large number of medicinal species are collected from these areas for commercial purpose and whole plant harvest makes the largest volume followed by seed, fruit, stem and tuber. The threat is more serious to the 9 IUCN listed species, of which root/rhizome/tuber is collected of 4, followed by stem and bark both of 2. These threatened species besides medicinal use also have several other uses including trade. It is frequently claimed that commercial utilisation of non-cultivated plant species in Nepal is unsustainable; although the scientific evidence found very weak empirical support for this. The traditional practice of Chepangs paid adequate attention to avoiding destructive harvesting. They used to leave some roots, tubers or bulbs for regeneration purposes but elder Chepangs said the high market demand and loss of customary rights induced uncontrolled harvest of open-access resources. Market driven problems like premature collection and unsustainable harvest induced by unhealthy competition from migrated people and increased collectors from neighbouring areas could affect resource base of this area. Unhealthy competition seems to be increased by market force and that could lead to extinction of species and when plant will be out of people's context the knowledge related to that will also disappears. Therefore, to protect species and their use knowledge it is important to control reckless harvest and this is only possible by enforcement of local social control mechanism. Besides, recognition of traditional knowledge by legitimising it to secure benefits related to it will encourage indigenous people to maintain traditional practices and protect natural resources.

KNOWLEDGE DISTRIBUTION

Several studies from all over the world indicate that elder people know more about plant use than younger and this corresponds to the findings of the present study. In Chepang communities also wild medicinal plants remain part of old people's context: they continue collection and preparation for utilisation.

Difference in knowledge between young and old people would be expected whereas significant difference between two adjacent age classes indicates problem of knowledge transmission. Loss of species, change in social practices, influence of migrated culture, influence of market, influence of development activities, change in life style, and policy problems are some of the important factors that potentially affect knowledge transmission. Knowledge generated by elders from historic practices and transmitted vertically to the younger generation is very much related to the affinity between family members. Traditionally, all members of a Chepang family used to gather around the fireplace in the morning and evening, where sharing of knowledge of various things including plant use took place. Multi-generational families provided ample opportunities for sharing indigenous knowledge and changes of such social structures affected knowledge transmission. Moreover, some of the species seems to be extinct locally and this might have affected knowledge in young people.

Knowledge is generated from observation and implementation, i.e. learning by doing. Women in rural societies worldwide are often primarily responsible for ensuring household food security, health and family continuity and due to that women are expected to be more rich than men in indigenous plant use knowledge. However, medicinal plant knowledge analysis indicated that medicinal plant use knowledge specifically the one used to cure illness of serious nature was limited to traditional healers only. Moreover, there is clear evidence that in the homogeneous ward, men are in general more knowledgeable than women while women were more knowledgeable than men in heterogeneous ward. The reason for men being more knowledgeable then women in homogeneous ward is due to big difference in knowledge about medicinal plant use, and one of the reason for this difference could be because all shaman-healers are men and do the 'serious' medicinal plant collection, while women concentrate on plants used for common and minor illnesses.

Men were more knowledgeable in the homogeneous community (Ward no. 3) than in heterogeneous community (ward 4) also indicates erosion of indigenous knowledge due to socio-economic influences. In Ward no. 4, Chepangs' lifestyle is socially and economically influenced by the in-migrated non-Chepangs and Stamm et al., 2004 hold that the influence of an introduced culture results in loss of knowledge. More than half of the population of Ward no. 4 is non-Chepang. Moreover, changes in life style and socio-economic status of people are reflected in a declining use of wild plants which ultimately affects the knowledge transfer. The influence of non-Chepangs on the life style of Chepangs was observed most outspoken among the younger generation. Devaluation of traditional plant use practices by non-Chepangs has developed a prestige feeling among them, making the young Chepangs embarrassed at collecting wild plant products and follow traditional practices in general, which resulted in loss of collection skills (e.g. tuber and root digging) and use knowledge. Some Chepangs have married non-Chepangs and due to that changed life style and cultural practices, and the interaction between children of the two groups has also changed the cultural and social understanding of Chepang children. Moreover, like in other aboriginal populations Christian missionaries made several young Chepangs stop practising traditional spiritual and cultural activities, including herbal treatment from *Pande* (healer) and non-Chepangs encouraged them to use modern medicine, leading to a loss of indigenous knowledge of medicinal plants.

14

Fauna Used in Popular Medicine in Northeast Brazil

BACKGROUND

Humans depend on biodiversity and the capacity of ecosystems to provide a multitude of goods and services that underpin a healthy human and natural environment. Biodiversity is essential for human health, for example, in the provision of the raw materials for medicines. Indeed, some 20,000 species are used in traditional medicine, which forms the basis of primary health care for about 80 percent of the 3 billion people in developing countries. More than half of the world's modern drugs are derived from biological resources, which supports the traditional and modern pharmaceutical sectors.

Plants and animals have been used as medicinal sources since ancient times, and even today animal and plant-based pharmacopeias continue to play an essential role in world health care. Although plants and plant-derived materials make up the majority of ingredients used in most traditional medical systems globally, whole animals, animal parts, and animal-derived products (e.g., urine, fat, etc.) also constitute important elements of the materia medica. Indeed, zootherapy, the use of animal products in healing, is an ancient and widespread practice across most cultures.

Animals have been broadly used since ancient times in Brazilian traditional medicine, and have played a significant role in healing practices. Expressions of traditional medicine in the country, particularly of zootherapy, represent an interaction of native, African and European elements, since the beginning of colonization, resulting in a rich ethnomedicine used by people belonging to different social classes in Brazil. Nevertheless, the use of animal species as remedies, although representing an important component of traditional medicine (sometimes in association with plant species), has been much less studied than medicinal plants in the country.

Little attention has been paid to the cultural, medical, economic, or ecological significance of zootherapeutic practices, even though the federal government's National Policy of Pharmaceuticals (Política Nacional de Medicamentos, Portaria no. 3916/98) specifies that "the support to research aiming to use the therapeutic potential of the national flora and fauna, with emphasis on certification of their medical properties, should be continued and expanded". Nevertheless, since the 1980s various publications have shown the importance of zootherapy for traditional communities from distinct socio-cultural-environmental landscapes in Brazil. Most of the available information on the subject is concentrated in the Northeast of the country.

In addition, the edibility of these medicinal resources must be analyzed because there must be complex interactions between diet and the medicinal use. A number of food animals are also used as remedies. Yet, our knowledge about the practice of food medicine is limited, particularly with regards to the traditional consumption of animal food-medicines. Although often regarded as supplementary to local peoples' diet, wild food and medicine are essential in times of crisis and play an important nutritional role. The neglect of traditional food and medicines may seriously deteriorate the health and well being of traditional peoples. Furthermore, nature-based traditional food and medicine are generally viewed as interchangeable, diet being highly regarded as the primary basis for sustaining and/or restoring health and well-being. Consequently, foods are considered and often times chosen for their distinctive medicinal or healing values. Given Brazil's significant cultural and biological diversity, the country can be used as a useful case study to increase our knowledge of faunistic resources used as medicines, and to draw attention to the need to protect traditional knowledge and biodiversity. In that context, the aim of this paper is summarize current knowledge on zootherapeutic practices in of Northeast of Brazil, based on information compiled from ethnobiological scientific literature, aiming to establish a regional data base. Contributions is expected in order to increase our knowledge concerning the faunistic resources used in the traditional medicine in the country, alerting for the need of protecting the biodiversity and the traditional knowledge and still emphasize the importance of a therapeutic modality that although widely disseminated at the country, is getting little attention from the scientific community.

METHODS

Study Area

The total area of the Brazilian Northeast is 1,561,177.8 km^2, which extends from 02°54 to 17°21S and from 35° to 46°30W and includes nine States: Maranhão, Piauí, Ceará, Rio Grande do Norte, Paraíba, Pernambuco, Alagoas, Sergipe and Bahia. This region is home to around 51 million people, representing 28.9% of the total population of Brazil, most of whom live in the urban area. The inhabitants of Northeast Brazil exhibit a high degree of race mixing. According to the 2006 census of Brazilian Institute for Geography and Statistics (IBGE), people of multiracial (European, Amerindian and African) background make up 62.5% of the population, while those of total or predominantly Black ancestry account for 7.8%. This region was not heavily affected by the wave of European immigration that took place in Southern Brazil during the 19th century – the Northeast was (and still is) the poorest part of Brazil, and therefore there was little incentive for new immigrants to stay.

As a result of the huge land mass involved, the diverse physio-geography of the region, as well as the conjunction of two major weather systems, provided by the NE and SE trade winds, rainfall patterns in Northeast Brazil are typically diverse and instable. The precipitation within the region varies from being extremely wet, with an annual rainfall of up to around 2,000 mm along the coast, to only 300–500 mm in the semi-arid zone, where the rainfall is usually restricted to a few months during the year. The availability of water determines the type and abundance of vegetation and fauna that exists in the region, as therefore in turn the patterns of human exploitation of natural resources.

The predominant vegetation type in this region is composed of several forms of caatinga biome. The structure of these forests can vary considerably from forests composed of mostly spiny trees, 6 to 10 m tall, often with a ground-layer of small deciduous shrubs and annual herbs, predominantly Leguminosae, to deciduous woodlands of lower stature, with a high proportion of shrubs and subshrubs and the presence of many cacti, bromeliads and Euphorbiaceae.

The Caatinga has been described as harboring relatively few species and having low numbers of endemic species. Some recent studies, however, have challenged this and demonstrated the importance of the region for the conservation of a significant component of Brazilian biodiversity. Inventories and assessments have, to date, recorded 932 vascular plant species, 187 bees, 240 fishes, 167 reptiles and amphibians, 62 families and 510 species of birds, and 148 mammal species. Levels of endemism vary from about 7% for mammals to 3% in birds and 57% in fishes. The Northeast region as a whole holds more types of vegetation than any other region in Brazil. In addition to the Caatinga biome, there are the Atlantic Rainforests, seasonal forests and inland mountain forests, *restinga* and shore dunes, mangroves, cerrados (savannah-like vegetation) and 'campos rupestres', all of which exhibit rich animal and plant biodiversity.

Data Collection

In order to examine the diversity of animals used in traditional medicine in Northeast of Brazil, all available references or reports of folk remedies based on animals sources were examined. 34 ethnobiological sources documenting the medicinal use of animals were analyzed. Only taxa that could be identified to species level were included in the data base. Scientific names were updated in accordance with the Integrated Taxonomic Information System's "Catalogue of Life: 2008 Annual Checklist". The conservation status of the animal species follows IUCN, Convention on International Trade in Endangered Species of Wild Fauna and Flora – CITES, Brazil's official list of endangered species, and the national list of species of aquatic invertebrates and fishes endangered, overexploited, or threatened by exploitation.

The reputed therapeutic effects and ailments treated were grouped into 20 categories based on the classification used by the Centro Brasileiro de Classificacão de Doenças (Brazilian Center for the Classification of Diseases), following Alves and Rosa.

Table 1. Categories of diseases treated with zootherapeutic remedies in Northeast Brazil, according to the Brazilian Centre of Diseases Classification and the number of species used per category.

Categories of diseases	**Number of medicinal animals**
Some infections and parasitic diseases	58
Respiratory system	132
Digestive system	38
Undefined illnesses	71
External causes of morbidity and mortality	45
Osteomuscular system and conjunctive tissue	71
Injuries, poisoning and other consequences of external causes	77
Urinogenital system	19
Circulatory system	64
Skin and subcutaneous tissue	44
Nervous system	27
Neoplasias (tumours)	12
Ear (middle and inner ear) and mastoid apophysis	32

Blood and haematopoeitic organs, and some disorders of the immune system	4
Pregnancy, parturition, and puerperium	7
Symptoms, signs, and abnormal findings from medical and laboratorial examination, not categorized in other part or section	9
Mental and behavioral perturbations	12
Diseases of the endocrine glands, metabolism and nutrition	3
Ophthalmological diseases	13
Congenital malformations, deformities and cromossomic abnormalities	2

RESULTS AND DISCUSSION

The review revealed that at least 250 animal species (178 vertebrates and 72 invertebrates) are used for medicinal purposes in Northeast of Brazil. The inventoried species comprise 10 taxonomic categories and belong to 141 Families. The groups with the greatest number of species were fishes (n = 58), mammals (n = 47) and reptiles (n = 37). These results are in line with previous studies carried out around the world, as numerous workers have pointed out that vertebrates are the animals most frequently used in folk medicine.

The number of medicinal species catalogued was quite expressive and demonstrate the importance of zootherapy as alternative therapeutic in Northeast of Brazil. Ethnobiological studies encompassing information on the medicinal use of biological resources cover 06 states: Paraíba, Piauí, Pernambuco, Alagoas, Maranhão and Bahia, the latter being state with the highest number of studies. No published accounts were found for the states of Ceará, Sergipe and Rio Grande do Norte. Due to the lack of studies in some states of Northeast Brazil, and to the fact that only taxa that could be identified to the species level were included in the review, is expected the number of medicinal animals to be greater than the 250 species compiled.

Of the 250 medicinal animal species which have been recorded, 175 (70%) were also used as food. The high number of animals used both as food and medicine is not surprising given the important role played by wildlife as a source of protein in different parts of the world. In at least 62 countries worldwide, wildlife (including fish) provides significant proteins, calories, and essential fats to rural communities. The extensive use of foods as medicinal remedies reported in our study is in line with recent field investigations around the world. The degree of overlap between medicinal and nutritional uses of wild animals observed in our study was high, and left no doubt about the importance of wild animals in human diets and healing activities.

Also, this work showed that exists a larger knowledge on medicinal animals in predominantly rural areas, nevertheless, also drew attention to the zootherapeuticals knowledge of the urban poor in cities across the Northeast region. The notable use and commercialization of medicinal animals to alleviate and cure health problems and ailments in the cities of Brazil reveals the resilience of that therapeutic alternative, in spite of the influence of the western medicine. In urban areas, the people brought from their villages to the cities much valuable knowledge on animals-based remedies that is rarely studied. The use of similar resources as medicines in more remote and urban areas suggest that zootherapeutic practices may function as a social conduit which, in conjunction with other factors, helps to maintain the connections between rural and peasant people living in cities and their own traditional culture and values. More specifically, it indicates the potential for exchange of materials and information on illnesses and treatments between more remote and urban communities.

Medicinal animals recorded can be used whole or in parts such as fat, flesh, bone, bone marrow, cartilage, skin, tail, feather, liver, bile ("fel"), milk, rattle (from rattlesnakes), spine, shell, honey, wax, scale, rostral expansion, otolith, penis, carapace, blood, gizzard, beak, cocoon, teeth, tongue, egg, egg shells, tibia, secretions, head, heart, urine, foot, leg, nest, guts, pollen, ear, spawn, nail, horn, sucking dish and eye. Similarly, the most of zootherapeutic resources used in Northeast of Brazil have been recorded in studies previous in others regions of country, and of the world.

Beyond the use for treating human diseases, zootherapeutical resources are also used in ethnoveterinary medicine. Barboza et al. recorded the utilization of animals (zootherapeutics) as sources of medicines in folk veterinary medicine (ethnoveterinary) in semiarid northeast region and verified that 15 animals are used in the prevention or cure of animals' illnesses in that region.

Distinct preparation and administration manners of the zootherapic resources are reported in the works, but in general, hard parts, such as teeth, nails, shells, rattles from snakes, fish scales, bone, and cartilage, generally are dried in the sun, grated, and crushed to powder, and then administered as tea or taken during meals. Fat, body secretions, and oil are either ingested or used as an ointment. Some animals are utilized in combination with plants and/or other animal species, constituting the ingredients of what the interviewees call "garrafadas" a concoction defined by Camargo and Ngokwey, as a therapeutic drink composed of various plants soaked in *cacha, ca* (Brazilian sugar cane liquor) or white wine and contained in a bottle (*garrafa* in portuguese, hence the name *garrafada*). The uses of medicinal plants and animals overlap in many cases, as might be expected, as phytotherapy and zootherapy are well known and widely used therapeutic alternatives in contemporary societies. Considering the fact that the use of medicinal animals and plants is quite common in most areas of Northeast Brazil, various overlapping usages might well be expected among traditional remedies.

The zootherapeutic resources recorded were used to treat different diseases. The most widely treated condition were asthma, rheumatism and sore throat, conditions, which had a wide variety of animals to treat them with. Many animals were used for the treatment of multiple ailments. The highest numbers of animal species (132, 52.8%) have been reported for the treatment of Respiratory system related problems. Injuries, poisoning and other consequences of external causes are treated with 77 species (30.8%). 71 (28.4%) animal species are reported in uses in Undefined illnesses category (that includes all citations for diseases with unspecific symptoms). Problems of osteomuscular system and conjunctive tissue are reported to be treated with 71 (28.8%) species. Circulatory system related problems are treated with 64 species (25.6%).

Sanitary conditions of the zootherapeutics products generally were poor with obvious contamination risks to these products. These observations point to the need for sanitary measurements to be taken with medicinal animal products and the importance of including considerations about zootherapy into public health programs. Although the need for implementation of sanitary measures to the trade of animal or their parts for medicinal purposes is evident, adoption of regulatory measures faces considerable challenges, among them ensuring adequate participation of all stakeholders involved, monitoring of the activity, and combating illegal, unreported and unregulated trade. Additionally, chemical and pharmacological studies are necessary in order to clarify the eventual therapeutic usefulness of this class of biological remedies. The possibility of using various remedies for the same ailment is popularly valued, as it renders an adaptation to the availability/accessibility of animals possible.

The economic and geographic accessibility of medicinal animals, perceived efficacy and sociocultural factors were main reasons for popularity of zootherapy. Because Brazil is highly heterogeneous socially and profoundly unequal in distribution of income, socioeconomic aspects play a role in the perseverance of zootherapeutic practices. For the majority of the population, access to hospital care is available within the public sector, but the organization of the health-care system reflects the schisms within Brazilian society: high-technology private care is available to the rich, but only inadequate public care is available to the poor, which makes the use of available, affordable animal and plant remedies an important alternative. The high number of species registered evidenciates that the animals are therapeutic resources culturally important.

Nevertheless, the lack of zootherapeutic studies in Brazil (and in the world in general) has contributed to an underestimation of the importance of zootherapeutic resources in this country. Alves and Rosa, suggest that one of the factors that certainly contribute to the information scarcity on the subject is the semi-clandestine or clandestine nature of the trade and use of medicinal animals, generally result in usuaries and traders being more resistant to provide information. The most of medicinal animals are wild and protected by law. Nevertheless, although Brazilian legislation forbids commercial use of wild fauna (Article 1 Law 5,197 January 3, 1967 and Article 29 of Law 9,605 February 12, 1998), medicinal products and derivatives made from animals are commonly traded in many Brazilian cities.

Most of the species used (*n* = 230; 92%) are wild caught. In most cases remedies were prepared from dead specimens. Many of the medicinal animals are of conservation concern. Many of the recorded species (52 out of 250) are on either the IUCN Red List of Threatened Species, CITES list (Convention on International Trade in Endangered Species of Wild Fauna and Flora, Brazil's official list of endangered species, or the National List of species of aquatic invertebrates and fishes endangered, overexploited or threatened by exploitation. These results demonstrate the need to assess the implications of the use and trade of animal used in traditional medicines on their wild populations.

As pointed out by Alves et al, there is a need to increase our understanding of the biology and ecology of species commonly used as remedies to better assess the impacts of harvesting them (for medicinal or other purposes) on their wild populations. Medicinal species whose conservation status is in question should receive urgent attention, and aspects such as habitat loss and alteration should be discussed in connection with present and future medicinal uses. As Anyinam remarked, environmental degradation affects users of traditional medicine both by limiting their access to the resources traditionally used and by diminishing the knowledge base in their community upon which traditional medicine is constructed. Studies on traditional uses of faunistic resources should be carried out with other links to conservation biology, public health policies, sustainable management of natural resources and biological prospection is of great importance.

CONCLUSION

A total of 250 animals are used for medicinal purposes in the Northeast of Brazil, evidencing that the zootherapy represents a traditional practice in the region. The high number of animal species registered reveals the cultural importance of that practice as therapeutic alternative, being occasionally used in association with medicinal plants. In a country like Brazil, where the majority of the population has no access modern allopathic medicines, local medicinal animals and plant knowledge systems is of significance. The population uses traditional medicine due to the relatively low cost of traditional medicine and difficult access to modern health facilities. Nevertheless, the interest in and intrinsic value of zootherapy not be only be attributed to the lack of access to modern medicinal services. Even in cities where modern health services are more accessible and specialized; many people continue to go to traditional healers showing the cultural acceptability of such practices. Besides the biological aspects, the economical and sociocultural factors influence the relationship of the local gathered people and the zootherapic resources usage. The need of new studies is evidenced which approach the medicinal fauna of Brazil, seeking for a better understanding of this therapy form, not only in its ecological aspects, but also cultural and pharmacological.

15

Cultural Transmission of Traditional Knowledge

Traditional ecological knowledge (TEK) entails intricate integration between human beings and their natural resources. This construct has been defined as the knowledge acquired by local communities through history, by means of direct experience and contact with nature. It comprises a wide spectrum of rural inhabitants' lives, which include material, spiritual and cultural traits such as wild plant knowledge or traditional agriculture. This cumulative body of knowledge and beliefs evolves by adaptive processes and is handed down through generations by cultural transmission. Therefore, this knowledge is a dynamic process, which generally responds in a flexible way to environmental and socio-cultural changes.

Cultural transmission is a process of social dissemination in which behaviour patterns, cosmological beliefs, the culture's technological knowledge, etc. are communicated and acquired. This way of transmission is not simple, and it depends on many factors, such as age, gender and other socio-cultural factors. Cultural transmission occurs between individuals of different generations but within genealogy (vertical transmission), as is the case from parent to child; and it may also occur between individuals of the same generation, irrespective of their relationship (horizontal or contagious transmission). It has been found that vertical transmission is highly conservative. That is why, with this type of transmission, innovations might be very slow to spread in the population unless other modes of cultural transmission are also employed. In the case of "one-towards-many" mode of transmission, communication is highly efficient and cultural change may be quite rapid. On the other hand, in "many-towards-one" way of transmission, an individual is assumed to be influenced by many transmitters, and all transmitters act in concert so that social influence is reciprocally reinforced.

Paths of cultural transmission can change during lifetime. It is well known that parents, who share their context with their children, play a crucial role in transmitting knowledge in early life. However, as time goes by, peers, who might come from different scenarios, become more significant. In addition, cultural learning also continues throughout adulthood, as individuals interact with new social contexts; an interesting issue which has received little attention. Furthermore, aside from the importance of social-dependent contexts in cultural transmission, individual idiosyncratic factors are also relevant in this acquisition process, most of which derive from personal experiences that promote active filtering of cultural input. Local communities such as the Mapuche have a particular concept of nature which could contribute to the development of sustainable management practices, promoting biological and socio-cultural diversity. There is an increasingly comprehensive appreciation of this knowledge and biodiversity conservation projects have been more successful when local knowledge was considered.

The Mapuche people were ancient inhabitants of the South Andean region, who lived as hunter-gatherers and semi nomadic horticulturists, in isolated and independent communities. Since the Spanish conquest, these populations have been undergoing severe changes, which dramatically modified their living conditions and caused processes of erosion of their cultural heritage. Among other customs, their health system, diet and horticultural knowledge greatly changed, altering their gathering and cultivating experience. In spite of these changes, the Mapuche people still maintain wild plant use and horticultural practices as important aspects of their cultural traditions.

Traditional ecological knowledge related to wild plant use has suffered significant transformations, such as the incorporation of exotic medicinal and edible species. At present, this gathering practice tends to be declining over generations. Young people tend to leave their homes, abandoning their ancestral customs as they refocus their interests on the demands of western culture.

In relation to their horticultural tradition, other changes have occurred. Native crops such as maize, quinoa, potatoes, pumpkin and pepper have decreased in use, while barley, wheat and oats have been included.

Nowadays, their horticultural practices are influenced by extension agent institutions such as INTA (National Institute of Agricultural Technology), PSA (Agricultural Social Program) and CIESA (Center of Investigation and Teaching of Sustainable Agriculture) which have introduced new crops and technologies. In contrast, wild plant gathering does not seem to be influenced so much by these extension institutions.

In the present study, we have compared the cultural transmission of two types of traditional ecological knowledge in two communities of North-western Patagonia.

In the Pilcaniyeu community, we studied the transmission of traditional knowledge related to horticultural practices in home-gardens, greenhouses and gardens, and compared with wild plant gathering in the Cuyin Manzano community.

Whereas, wild plant gathering is a frequent custom among these rural inhabitants and has been thoroughly studied, horticultural practice has not been previously explored in the region. Both traditions had been historically important for sustenance and are still scenarios for transmission of ancient knowledge, that is why the comparison between both could shed interesting information.

We have analysed the actors involved in social networks associated with this learning process, investigating at what life history phase plant knowledge is learned, modes of transmission, and who the principal transmitters were in childhood and adulthood.

METHODS

Study Sites

The Pilcaniyeu community is located in the province of Rio Negro, Argentina (41° 7'S and 70° 44'W), and has approximately 1445 inhabitants. Pilcaniyeu's nearest urban population is Bariloche, located 75 km away. The area has a mean annual temperature of 7.3°C and a mean annual precipitation of 264.80 mm. It is characterized by the Patagonian steppe ecosystem, where sandy soils are dominant and the vegetation cover is mostly composed of shrubs and herbs: neneo (*Mulinum spinosum*), charcao (*Senecio filaginoides*); coirón amargo (*Stipa humilis*, *Stipa speciosa*) and *Poa huecu*, *Bromus macranthus*, *Poa ligularis*, *Festuca argentina* and other herbs.

It is also characterized by valleys and swamp areas, with rocky patches in other sectors. The economic sustenance of most inhabitants is cattle-raising, but some work as employees of public institutions and practice horticulture as well. Since 1992, extension agents such as INTA, have been in charge of promoting family, community and school home-gardens in Pilcaniyeu, Ñorquinco and Bariloche. They have been working with rural residents to help agro-systems and encourage socioeconomic development in their communities. In order to promote horticulture, extension agents have introduced new technology, practices and knowledge. As an example of new technology, they have provided the materials to build greenhouses and tools necessary for horticultural practice. These were considered as new technology, given that greenhouses were not traditionally developed by their ancestors. Furthermore, they periodically distribute seeds of exotic plants such as lettuce, carrot, chard, melon, etc. and visit the people to provide assistance according to their agricultural needs.

The Cuyin Manzano is an small rural community made up of 18 families, which is located in the Nahuel Huapi National Park (40° 45 S and 71° 10 W), Neuquén, Argentina, 80 km away from Bariloche city. This location is in a transition forest, dominated by a conifer species, *Austrocedrus chilensis*, with the presence of the deciduous species *Nothofagus pumilio*, at higher elevations and *N. antarctica* in the underbrush and scrubs. This area has a mean annual temperature between 5.4° and 9.5°C. Cattle-raising and handicrafts are the principal economic activities of most inhabitants.

Both populations are of mestizo origin, some inhabitants are direct descendants of the Mapuche people, while others have mixed ancestry. At present Pilcaniyeu and Cuyín Manzano have both lost their traditional Mapuche roots, i.e., the inhabitants do not speak the Mapuche language (Mapudumgun), and they have lost their political leaders (caciques) and shamans (machis).

Cuyín Manzano's social organization is weak; the primary school is the most significant communal structure. Pilcaniyeu, on the other hand, shows a more intricate social and political organization. There are several communal structures such as primary and secondary schools, a Town Hall, a local Hospital, and other facilities related to cultural, social, recreational and community development.

ETHNOBOTANICAL DATA COLLECTION

Ethonobotanical information was compared using data from fieldwork done in Pilcaniyeu and from a previous study done in Cuyin Manzano. Both ethnographic studies are really comparable given that all methodological procedures were followed in the same way, in spite of the fact that the topics surveyed differed. With the intention of developing the proposed objectives, a formal presentation was initially made to the authorities of each community to request their consent to work in the area. Moreover, in each visited domestic unit, we asked for voluntary participation in our interview. Ethnobotanical fieldwork was conducted by means of semi-structured interviews in the summer of 2001 in Cuyín Manzano and in the summer of 2007 in Pilcaniyeu. In both communities, participants were randomly selected, each representing a different family. A total of 30 people (20 women and 10 men) between 18 and 85 years old, were interviewed in the Pilcaniyeu community (approximately representing 20% of the total number of families), specifically those who dedicate greater time to horticultural practices.

A total of 16 individuals (7 women and 9 men) between 27 and 74 years old were interviewed in Cuyín Manzano (representing 80% of the total number of families). The semi-structured interviews, which lasted approximately 60 to 90 minutes, were based on general aspects of the interviewee's daily life in relation to plants. In the community of Pilcaniyeu, we asked about cultivated plants and traditional horticultural practices, while in the community of Cuyin Manzano we investigated wild plant knowledge and gathering practices. The interviewees' personal data, such as gender and age, was gathered as well. We were also interested in aspects related to cultural transmission of traditional knowledge: at what age and how plant knowledge was learned and who the principal transmitters were. In order to prepare field herbariums, wild plants and cultivated species were collected in both communities with the participation of the inhabitants which were visited in a second opportunity. The recorded registers, field notebooks, photographic material and field herbariums were deposited in the Ecotono Laboratory, Centro Regional Universitario Bariloche. Nomenclature follows Correa, Marticorena & Quesada and Ezcurra & Brion.

DATA ANALYSIS

In both communities, the following aspects related to cultural transmission were categorized: at what life history phase plant knowledge was learned, modes of transmission and who the principal transmitters were in childhood and adulthood. In turn, the frequencies of each category for each question were obtained. Additionally, in order to quantify the richness related to both practices, we calculated the total number of species recorded in each community. The frequency of these categories was analysed with the Chi-square test of independence ($p < 0.05$).

RESULTS

Modes of Transmission in Childhood

In the Pilcaniyeu community, the dwellers mentioned different transmitters of traditional knowledge related to horticultural practices and that they have learnt about these practices since childhood. When we compared the categories mentioned, significant differences were found among their responses ($X^2_5 = 16.424$, $p < 0.05$). Both parents were mentioned as main transmitters of this type of knowledge (39%). However, mothers seem to be important transmitters since they were mentioned in second place (22.2%); followed by grandmothers (11.1%). On the other hand, in 8.3% of the cases, learning was cited from their fathers. In only one case, a grandfather was mentioned as the first transmitter (2.8%). Additionally, in 5.5% of the cases other relatives (aunt, mother-in-law, etc.) were mentioned. The whole family was also mentioned as the source of learning in 5.5% of the cases. Finally, the same proportion was recorded for extra-family learning (teachers, friends, etc.).

In Cuyín Manzano, the informants mentioned different people as transmitters and that they have learnt about wild plant gathering practice in childhood as well. When these categories were compared, significant differences were found ($X^2_4 = 17.81$, $p = 0.001$). This traditional practice seems to be mainly transmitted by interviewee's mothers, and grandmothers were specifically mentioned by 50% of the cases when grandparents were cited.

MODES OF TRANSMISSION IN ADULTHOOD

Significant differences were found in terms of who the main transmitters were in this analysis in the community of Pilcaniyeu ($X^2_3 = 12{,}939$, $p < 0\text{-}05$). In 43.5% of the cases, we observed that adult informants do not consult other people, which means that they learn about horticulture through personal experience. Local people ("locals") represent an important source of learning (28%). This category corresponds to those inhabitants of Pilcaniyeu with vast experience in horticultural practices, an inherited tradition in their families, who have lived in the region for a long time. Extension agents, such as INTA or PSA, were also mentioned as important transmitters, but in a smaller proportion (18%). They have introduced new practices and technology, such as the use of greenhouses, which differ from the traditional knowledge of local people. Finally, in 10% of the cases, adult informants consult their family.

More than half of the families (68.6%) have incorporated the use of greenhouses. Sixty percent of the informants received help from extension agents (PSA and INTA), while the other 40% built their greenhouses by their own means, with the aid of other family members, neighbours, etc. It seems that this new practice is spread by horizontal transmission among local dwellers.

Traditional knowledge related to wild plant gathering practice in the community of Cuyin Manzano is acquired mostly through vertical transmission which prevails throughout informants' lives. Horizontal and oblique (one-toward-many or many to one) modes of transmissions were not documented in this community.

Plant Species Utilized and Common Uses in Both Populations

In Pilcaniyeu, 124 ethnospecies were recorded: 75 in home-gardens, 63 in greenhouses and 68 in gardens. Most species (113 spp.) were exotic, which means that they came from other biogeographic regions; while 11 were native to Patagonia. It is important to mention that some of these native species, such as *Chenopodium ambrosioides* and *Anarthorphyllum rigidum*, are not specifically cultivated but tolerated as part of the cultivated areas. Most species were cultivated for edible purposes (home consumption) (41%); whereas 28% were mentioned for ornamental purposes and 20% were cited for medicinal use.

Plant species collected in home-gardens, greenhouses and gardens utilized by Pilcaniyeu people

Botanic Family			
	Common name	*Scientific name*	Origin
Amaryllidaceae			
	Narcizo	*Narcissus* sp.	Exotic
Anacardiaceae			
	Molle	*Schinus o´donellii* Barkley	Native

Apiaceae		
Apio	*Apium graveolens* L.	Exotic
Cilantro	*Coriandrum sativum* L.	Exotic
Hinojo	*Foeniculum vulgare* Mill.	Exotic
Perejil	*Petroselinum crispum* (Mill.) Nym.	Exotic
Perejil crespo	*Petroselinum crispum* var. *crispum* (Mill.) Airy-Shaw	Exotic
Zanahoria	*Daucus carota* var. *sativa* L.	Exotic
Araliaceae		
Hiedra	*Hedera helix* L.	Exotic
Araucariaceae		
Araucaria	*Araucaria araucana* (Mol.) K. Koch	Native
Asteraceae	*Taraxacum officinale* Web.	Exotic
Achicoria		
Ajenjo	*Artemisia absinthium* L.	Exotic
Caléndula	*Calendula officinalis* L.	Exotic
Carqueja	*Baccharis sagittalis* (Less.) DC.	Native
Chilca	*Baccharis salicifolia* (Ruiz & Pav.) Pers.	Native
Coqueta	*Bellis perennis* L.	Exotic
Éter	*Artemisia abrotanum* L.	Exotic
Girasol enano	*Helianthus tuberosus* L.	Exotic
Lechuga	*Lactuca sativa* L.	Exotic
Manzanilla	*Chrysanthemum parthenium* (L). Bernhardi	Exotic
Margarita	*Chrysanthemum sp.*	Exotic
Margarita	*Matricaria inodora* L.	Exotic
Milenrama	*Achillea millefolium* L.	Exotic
Palma	*Tanacetum vulgare* L.	Exotic
Yerba de San Juanmenta extranjera o turca	*Tanacetum balsamita* L.	Exotic
Brassicaceae		
Alelí	*Cheirantus cheiri* L.	Exotic
Matuerzo	*Coronopus didymus* (L.) Smith	Exotic
Nabiza	*Brasicca napus* var. *arvensis* f. *annus* (Schubl. et Mart.) Thell	Exotic
Nabo	*Brassica rapa* L.	Exotic
Rabanito	*Raphanus sativus* L.	Exotic

Repollo	*Brassica oleraceae* var. *capitata* L.	Exotic
Repollo corazón de buey	*Brassica oleraceae* L.	Exotic
Buddlejaceae		
Pañil	*Buddleja araucana* Phil.	Native
Caprifoliaceae		
Sauco	*Sambucus nigra* L.	Exotic
Caryophyllaceae		
Clavel	*Dianthus caryophyllus* L.	Exotic
Celastraceae		
Maitén	*Maytenus boaria* Molina	Native
Chenopodiaceae		
Acelga	*Beta vulgaris* var. *cicla* L.	Exotic
Espinaca	*Spinacia oleracea* L.	Exotic
Paico	*Chenopodium ambrosioides* L.	Native
Remolacha	*Beta vulgaris* var. *rapacea* L.	Exotic
Crassulaceae		
Rochela	(?)	Exotic
Cucurbitaceae		
Melón	*Cucumis melo* L.	Exotic
Pepino	*Cucumis sativus* L.	Exotic
Zapallito	*Cucurbita maxima* var. *zapallito* (Carr.) Millán	Exotic
Zapallito zuchini	*Cucurbita pepo* convar. *giromontiina* Duch	Exotic
Zapallo	*Cucurbita pepo* L.	Exotic
Elaeagnaceae		
Olivillo	*Elaeagnus angustifolia* L.	Exotic
Enoteraceae		
Clarquea	*Clarkia elegans* Dougl.	Exotic
Godesia	*Godetia* sp.	Exotic
Fabaceae		
Alfalfa	*Medicago sativa* L.	Exotic
Arveja	*Pisum sativum* L.	Exotic
Chocho	*Lupinus arboreus* Sims.	Exotic
Clarín	*Lathyrus latifolius* L.	Exotic
Haba	*Vicia faba* L.	Exotic
Monte guanaco	*Anarthrophyllum rigidum* (Gilies ex Hook. & Arn.) Hieron.	Native

Paramela	*Adesmia boronioides* Hook.f.	Native
Poroto	*Phaseolus* sp.	Exotic
Retama	*Cytisus scoparius* L. (Link.)	Exotic
Vicia	*Vicia* sp.	Exotic
Geraniaceae		
Malvón	*Pelargonium* sp.	Exotic
Lamiaceae		
Albahaca	*Ocimum basilicum* L.	Exotic
Lavanda	*Lavandula* sp.	Exotic
Malva rubia	*Marrubium vulgare* L.	Exotic
Menta blanca	*Mentha rotundifolia* (L.) Huds.	Exotic
Menta negra	*Mentha spicata* L.	Exotic
Orégano	*Origanum vulgare* L.	Exotic
Chascudo	*Origanum* (?)	Exotic
Poleo	*Mentha pulegium* L.	Exotic
Romero	*Rosmarinus officinalis* L.	Exotic
Salvia	*Salvia officinalis* L.	Exotic
Té del gato	*Nepeta cataria* L.	Exotic
Tomillo	*Thymus vulgaris* L.	Exotic
Toronjil	*Melisa officinalis* L.	Exotic
Lauraceae		
Laurel	*Laurus nobilis* L.	Exotic
Liliaceae		
Ajo	*Allium sativum* L.	Exotic
Ajo puerro	*Allium porrum* L.	Exotic
Cebolla	*Allium cepa* L.	Exotic
Cebolla de verdeo	*Allium fistulosum* L.	Exotic
Cebollita	*Allium* sp.	Exotic
Chalota	*Allium schoenoprasum* L.	Exotic
Tulipán	*Tulipa* sp.	Exotic
LinaceaeLino	*Linum usitatissimum* L.	Exotic
Malvaceae		
Malva	*Malva sylvestris* L.	Exotic
Malvón	*Althaea officinalis* L.	Exotic
OleaceaeLila	*Syringa vulgaris* L.	Exotic

Papaveraceae		
Amapola	*Papaver rhoeas* L.	Exotic
Celedonia	*Chelidonium majus* L.	Exotic
Copa de oro	*Eschscholtzia californica* Cham.	Exotic
Pinaceae		
Pino	*Pinus* sp.	Exotic
Plantaginaceae		
Llantén	*Plantago lanceolata* L.	Exotic
Poaceae		
Maíz	*Zea mays* L.	Exotic
Poa	*Poa* sp	?
Polygonaceae		
Ruibarbo	*Rheum rhabarbarum* L.	Exotic
Ranunculaceae		
Espuela de caballero o Pajarito	*Consolida ajacis* (L.) Schur	Exotic
Rosaceae		
Cerezo	*Prunus avium* L.	Exotic
Ciruelo	*Prunus domestica* L.	Exotic
Corona de novia	*Spiraea lanceolata* Poir.	Exotic
Duraznero	*Prunus persica* L. Batsch	Exotic
Frambuesa	*Rubus idaeus* L.	Exotic
Frutilla	*Fragaria vesca* L.	Exotic
Guindo	*Prunus cerasus* L.	Exotic
Manzano	*Malus domestica* Borkh	Exotic
Membrillo	*Cydonia oblonga Mill.*	Exotic
Níspero	*Mespilus germanica* L.	Exotic
Rosa	*Rosa* sp.	Exotic
Rutaceae		
Naranjo	*Citrus sinensis* L.	Exotic
Ruda	*Ruta graveolens* L.	Exotic
Salicaceae		
Álamo	*Populus nigra* L.	Exotic
Álamo plateado	*Populus alba* L.	Exotic
Sauce	*Salix* sp.	Exotic

Saxifragaceae		
Casis	*Ribes* sp.	Exotic
Corinto	*Ribes aureum* Pursh.	Exotic
Grosella	*Ribes grossularia* L.	Exotic
Zarzaparrilla	*Ribes magellanicum* Poir.	Native
Scrophulariaceae		
Conejito	*Antirrhinum majus* L.	Exotic
Solanaceae		
Morrón	*Capsicum annuum* L.	Exotic
Papa	*Solanum tuberosum* L.	Exotic
Tomate	*Lycopersicum esculentum* var. *esculentum* Mill.	Exotic
Ulmaceae		
Olmo	*Ulmus* sp.	Exotic
Urticaceae		
Ortiga	*Urtica dioica* L.	Exotic
Verbenaceae		
Retamo	*Diostea juncea* (Gillies & Hook) Miers.	Native
Violaceae		
Pensamiento	*Viola tricolor* L.	Exotic
Vitaceae		
Uva	*Vitis vinifera* L.	Exotic

On the other hand, in Cuyín Manzano, 87 species were recorded, of which 47 were native and 40 exotic. Of the total number of species, 63 (72%) were cited for medicinal use and 24 (28%) were mentioned for edible purposes.

Discussion

In the present study we have found that traditional ecological knowledge related to horticultural practice and wild plant gathering is still transmitted over generations in rural populations of North-western Patagonia.

In the case of the Pilcaniyeu community, the transmission of traditional knowledge related to horticultural practices begins in the early stages of childhood, when accompanying their parents to cultivate the land. In this family tradition, women seem to play a predominant role. This knowledge is mostly transmitted vertically through family dissemination. In the Cuyin Manzano community, wild plant gathering is transmitted by family members during childhood as well.

Vertical transmission is the main mode of acquiring this traditional knowledge. Mothers are the first mentioned as principal transmitters, this fundamental role of women has also been found in other studies.

For example, it has been observed that wild fruit gathering is an activity mainly conducted by women, who transmit not only their traditional knowledge but also certain values of respect and connection with nature, generation after generation.

Similarly, women are generally the ones in charge of home-gardens, as well as of the transmission of traditional knowledge related to horticultural practices (e.g. following moon cycles, elaboration of natural herbicides, collection of seeds). Moreover, other studies emphasize female participation in projects destined to sustainable management practices in forests, due to their thorough knowledge of the area.

In Pilcaniyeu, people recognized and valued their personal experience related to horticultural practices. However, horizontal transmission is relevant at present, i.e. horticultural learning continues during adulthood.

At this life time, which has significant extra-familiar contributions, locals interchange knowledge and practices, probably relearning and changing their previously acquired information. This knowledge may or may not agree with what they learnt as a family tradition.

Horizontal mode of transmission related to home-garden management was also observed in other communities. Moreover, extension agents have introduced new practices and technology through a "one-toward-many" mode of transmission. According to Boesch & Tomasello cultural innovations may be rapidly incorporated by a community when these are introduced by an influential group.

This could be the case of the Pilcaniyeu community where extension agents might have initiated cultural changes on horticultural practices. The use of greenhouses was first introduced as a new technology by extension agents, and afterwards it spread among locals through horizontal transmission.

This could be an example of multiple sources of information and knowledge which coexist within a group, suggesting diverse ways of unfolding social learning processes.

The fact that horizontal transmission was not conspicuously detected in Cuyin Manzano could be related to methodological biases associated with self-report means of inquiry.

When interviews rely on self-reports, it is possible that informants tend to overemphasize the role of parents in acquiring ethnobotanical knowledge. During childhood, this knowledge is learned through vertical transmission although, later in life, locals often acquire extra-familiar information without being conscious of this process.

This might have also occurred in the Pilcaniyeu community in spite of the overt influence received from outsiders. Therefore, horizontal inputs might have been underestimated in the collected data, an issue that should be kept into consideration. As an example, they minimized the importance of external agents in the interviews, although most of families have incorporated greenhouses provided by them.

The incorporation of new practices and technology, which could lead to innovative processes, could also imply the loss of traditional ecological knowledge. At the same time, it could allow for the integration of new and ancestral practices, generating hybrid knowledge.

This process might indicate a dynamic response to their changing living conditions, suggesting local capacity for building social-ecological resilience. Resilience implies the capacity for learning and adapting. This process might be occurring in Pilcaniyeu, given that

68.6% of the families incorporated greenhouse, thus integrating their ancestral knowledge with new technologies and knowledge. Furthermore, the cultivation of exotic species and the replacement of native ones, which started with the Spanish Conquest, has become a long standing practice that still occurs nowadays. This process, which began in the Mapuche ancestral habitat, the forest, appears to have been enhanced in this new arid context, with the incorporation, for example, of greenhouses. This might indicate further adaptive possibilities.

Moreover, in Cuyin Manzano resilience could also be observed in relation to wild exotic species gathering. Though wild exotic plants were observed many years ago in this region, the relatively high proportion of non native species use could also be indicating a longstanding process of change. Both local practices, i.e. wild plant gathering and horticulture, are undergoing several transformations, showing the influences of environmental changes and cultural transmission.

Both wild plant gathering and horticultural practices imply personal connections with nature that might provide opportunities for learning, encouraging the development of attitudes which are associated with the protection of the environment. At present, there are fewer opportunities, especially for children, to spend time with and learn from parents, grandparents and others who are knowledgeable about conservation practices and beliefs, in addition to the introduction of schooling into family life. Local knowledge is remembered through social memory, which describes how an individual thought or observation can become part of the collective knowledge of a group, so as to allow communal understanding of environmental change and the transmission of experience.

CONCLUSION

In order to preserve traditional ecological knowledge, it would be convenient to generate connectedness within networks and groups so as to encourage vertical and horizontal transmission of traditional practices among locals. Therefore, it could be useful to bring back these results to the rural people and to promote community participation activities tending to share traditional knowledge such as workshops, field trips and seed interchange. This could enable greater integration between local and scientific knowledge, allowing for cultural and biological diversity.

For this purpose, it would also be necessary to create new mechanisms of communication between locals and western Institutions tending to facilitate better comprehension and self respect. In this way, investigations such as the present study could help by forming a bridge between local dwellers and extension agents who want to promote rural development. We consider that being receptive to local people's traditional ecological knowledge is important in order to generate more efficient aid to rural communities, as well as fostering western culture.

16

The Use of Magical Plants

Although the use of plants for treating supernaturally caused illnesses (e.g., soul loss, evil wind, witchcraft) has been documented in the Ecuador highlands, so-called magical plants have received much less focused attention than plants used for treating naturalistic disorders. Drawing on interviews done in 2002 and 2003 with 116 curanderos residing in the Ecuador highlands, this paper examines the characteristics of plants identified as magical, how they are used, and how the study of magical plants provides insights into the mindscape of residents of the highlands.

BACKGROUND

Traditional medical practitioners in the Ecuador highlands, those generically known as curanderos but especially the *limpiadores* ("cleaners"), make extensive use of magical plants in the treatment of supernatural folk illnesses such as *susto*, *mal viento, mal prójimo*, and *mal aire.* In most documentations on magical plant use over the past thirty or so years, however, the rationale underlying the use of magical plants is poorly described or not addressed at all. This paper reports on information gathered from 116 curanderos in the Ecuador highlands on the use of magical plants for healing. Topics discussed include the characteristics of plants identified as magical, why and how they are used for the treatment of selected folk illnesses, and finally how the study of magical plants provides insights into the worldview of highland residents.

METHODS

Residents of the Ecuador highlands have a wide variety of plants available for healing. Physiographically, the highlands are defined by two volcanic mountain ranges running from north to south. The botanical diversity of the region reflects in large measure variation in elevation: an inter-Andean valley of agricultural plots and pastures; lower montane rain forests and upper montane cloud forests on the mountain slopes; dry valleys in the south; and high altitude grass and desert *paramos* (plateaus).

Table: Province residence of curanderos

Province	Number	Percentage
Bolivar	85	73.00
Chimborazo	10	8.60
Cotopaxi	3	2.50
Imbabura	1	.80
Los Rios	6	5.10
Pinchincha	1	.80
Tungurhua	10	8.62
Totals	116	100.00

Informant interviews were done in 2002 and 2003 as part of a more encompassing investigation on the role of curanderos in the region's informal health care delivery system. Published sources on ethnomedicine in the Ecuador highlands and the Andean region were used to develop an interview schedule to gather baseline information on: (1) recruitment to the curandero role, (2) years of service, (3) client load, (4) articulation with and attitude toward the formal health care system, (5) types of services rendered and healing specializations, (6) types of folk illnesses recognized and treated, (7) therapeutic methods and *materia medica* used in the treatment of folk illnesses, and (8) types of curanderos. The interview schedule was pre-tested with 14 informants and subsequently underwent minor modifications. The investigation was also informed by numerous unscheduled interviews with residents of various communities in the highlands and first-hand observation of ritual healings. This paper reports on information related to items six and seven on the interview schedule.

Initially, informants were recruited opportunistically through co-author Alban's contacts in the Bolivar and Chimborazo Provinces. Recruitment of informants proved difficult in the more isolated highlands communities due the authors' outsider status and their likely perceived identification with the government and the related concern of being reported for practicing medicine without a license. To overcome these and other recruitment problems, we solicited the assistance of second-year nursing students enrolled at the Universidad Estatal de Bolivar located in Guaranda. Our reasoning was that the students would be familiar with curanderos in their native communities and, more important, that the curanderos would be more inclined to do an interview with a resident of their community than with an outsider. At a meeting with the nursing students in 2003 a presentation was given by co-author Albán and the director of the university's nursing program on the purpose and scope of the project.

The interview schedule and interviewing techniques were discussed later in classes with the students. The students were asked to identify and interview one curandero in their local community as a course assignment. Each student was given one dollar to cover transportation expenses. All informant responses were recorded directly on the interview schedule in Spanish. All the interviews, which on average lasted a little more than an hour, were done in the informants' homes. Since many informants were illiterate or marginally literate, written informed consent was not obtained. All informants, however, were orally informed of the purpose of the research and assured of the confidentiality of their identity. Not surprisingly, some students were much more successful than others doing the interview, and some informants were more prodigious and reflective in their responses than others. Eight interviews were withdrawn because the informants provided little or no information;

four other interviews were withdrawn because they were informant duplicates.

Sixty-six (56.9%) of the curanderos were male, 50 (43.1%) were female. Of the 108 informants who reported their age, the range of age was 25 to 87 with an average age of 54. The majority (n = 67, 62%) were in the 40 to 59 age group; 10 were in the 20 to 39 age group. Years of service as a curandero ranged from 2 to 55 years with an average period of service of 21.57 years. Clients served by the informants per week ranged from 2 to 200 with an average client load of 21.9. Information on the level of educational attainment was obtained from 112 informants. Fifty-seven percent (n = 64) had completed primary school. Sixteen percent (n = 18) attended but did not complete primary school, and of these individuals 16 went no further than the fourth grade. Twenty-two percent (n = 25) were illiterate. Two informants completed high school and only one had a university degree. All the informants resided in rural communities, ranging from rural hamlets to small towns.

The largest town represented in the study, Guaranda, has a population of about 5,000. Reflecting the rural economy of the highlands, the majority of the male informants worked as farmers or manual laborers. The female informants were mainly housewives, and most of them were actively involved in family farming activities. Some informants, both males and females, earned income through selling herbs, produce, animals and animal products, handicrafts, cooked foods, and merchandise at local town markets. If the client loads reported by the informants are valid, many curanderos enhanced their income considerably from their healing work. Some of their services are expensive.

The performance of the *limpieza*, a cleansing ritual discussed later, can be, depending on a client's condition, depleting, costing as much as $25.00 according to some reports, and this does not include the cost of materia medica (e.g., cigarettes, cologne, plants, eggs, guinea pig) which in most cases the client is expected to bear. But even a few dollars is a lot for poor campesinos.

As noted previously, all the informants were *limpiadores*, but many of them reported providing other much sought after services. Some informants were highly knowledgeable herbalists; some were *sobadores* (massage therapists); some were skilled at magically dealing with various social problems such as helping people with unfaithful husbands and wives, casting love spells, obtaining employment, finding lost objects, and assisting students with performing well on exams by magically treating their textbooks. Some informants, mainly but not exclusively females, also served as *parteras* (midwives). One informant served as a *llamador* ("caller"), a healer who calls (i.e. retrieves) a departed soul back to an individual's body. The only type of curandero role not represented in the informant population is the shaman which we define as an individual who enters an altered state of consciousness to communicate with spirit beings. Shamans are present in the highlands, but are better represented in the Oriente (eastern rainforest) section of Ecuador.

Ethnicity in the highlands, which revolves around *mestizo*, *indígena* (indigenous, "Indian") and *blanco* (white) identities, is a sensitive and sometimes inflammatory topic for some residents. For this reason, information on ethnic self-identification was obtained only from informants who were friends or acquaintances of co-author Albán which amounted to 14. Eight self-identified as *mestizos*, 6 as *indígenas*. We compared the magical plants reported by the 12 *mestizo* curanderos with those reported by the 6 *indígena* curanderos and found a close correspondence in magical plants usage. Based on this admittedly limited comparison, we would predict that the belief in magical plants is a cultural tradition shared by both ethnic groups. A much more nuanced investigation, of course, might locate significant differences along ethnic lines.

RESULTS AND DISCUSSION

The information on magical plants presented here is based on a content analysis of informant responses to the sections of the interview schedule concerning the types of folk illnesses recognized and related therapeutic methods and materia medica used to treat them. The analysis revealed the use of 48 plants and a variety of other materia medica for the treatment of *mal aire/mal viento, espanto/susto, brujería, duende,* and *mal prójimo.* This discussion, however, is confined to those plants (n = 17, 35%) that had a frequency of response of three or more.

These plants and their uses are shown in Table below. Unfortunately, no voucher specimens of the plants were collected. The scientific names for the plants in Table below were derived from cross-checking vernacular names with scientific names in four sources. Final determination of the scientific name is based on *The Catalogue of Vascular Plants in Ecuador.* The lack of identified voucher specimens, of course, presents problems in terms of determining accurately the correspondence of use of plants among the curandero informants. Furthermore, we were unable to infer from the vernacular names the taxanomical classification of two plants listed on Table below (manchari and tigresillo).

Mal Aire/Mal Viento

Two authorities on ethnomedicine in Latin American observe that "airs" is "among the most elusive of illness concepts". Our investigation aligns with this observation. A few informants (n = 8) defined *mal aire* (bad air) as a naturalistic illness in terms of the hot/cold theory of illness causation. As they explained it, breathing in cold night air, moving rapidly from a warm to a cold ambient environment, or working up a sweat and not allowing for a proper cooling down period causes illness.

The majority of informants, however, defined *mal aire* in supernatural terms. As for *mal viento* (bad or evil wind), several informants (n = 46, 39.6%) reported that the terms *mal aire* and *mal viento* are interchangeable and refer to the same kind of supernaturally caused illness. Although some informants recognized *mal aire* and *mal viento* as two distinct supernatural folk illnesses in terms of causation or symptoms, the definitional criteria used by some informants to distinguish *mal aire* were the very same criteria used by other informants to define *mal viento.*

Table: Magical plants used by curanderos

Scientific Name	Reports	Part Used	Treatment Methods
Ambrosia arborecens Mill. Asteraceae	52	whole plant; leaves stems	brush body with whole plant; infusion made from leaves ingested
Baccharis latifolia (Ruiz & Pav) Pers	13	whole plant	brush body
Brugmansia sanguinea (Ruiz & Pav.) D. Don Solanaceae	8	leaves flowers	brush body with leaves and flowers
Citrus medica L. Rutaceae	6	fruit/rind	rub body with whole fruit or rind
Dianthus caryophyllus L. Caryophyllaceae	12	flowers	patient soaked in warm bath of flowers or sprayed with decoction of flowers
Eucalyptus globulus Labill. Myrtaceae	17	leaves stems	brush body with small branches or vaporization of leaves
Mentha × piperita L. Lamiaceae	7	leaves	infusion ingested
Minthostachys mollis (Kunth) Griseb Lamiaceae	55	whole plant	brush body with whole plant
Nicotiana tabacum L. Solanaceae	50	leaves	smoke from cigarette blown on patient; also used to diagnose presence of *mal* (negative energy)
Prunus serotina Ehrh. Rosaceae	4	leaves stems	brushing with leaves
Rosmarinus officinalis L. Lamiaceae	12	leaves stems	brush body with leaves; infusion made from leaves and stems ingested

Ruta graveolens L. Rutaceae	65	whole plant; leaves, flowers	brush with leaves; more rarely, patient soaked in warm bath of leaves and/or flowers
Tanacetum parthenium L. Sch. Bip Asteraceae	46	whole plant	brush with whole plant
Urtica dioica L. Urticaceae	14	whole plant; leaves	brush with whole plant; infusion made from leaves ingested
Valeriana decussate Ruiz & Pav. Valerianaceae	6	leaves	infusion made from leaves ingested
Unknown	8	whole plant	brush body with whole plant
Unknown	3	whole plant	brush body with whole plant

The underlying supernatural meaning of *mal aire/mal viento* is the existence of a malevolent, destructive force or power that is transmitted through the air and wind. Following the discourse of some informants and McKee, we use the term *mal* in reference to this malevolent power. As observed by McKee in her study of diarrheal illness in the highlands, *mal* is in one sense animatistic, an impersonal force similar to the Melanesian concept of *mana*. Informants reported that *mal aire/mal viento* illness is caused by a person's exposure to *mal* at certain locales that they described as *lugares pesados* or *lugares malignos* (heavy or malignant places). These places include unpopulated areas, abandoned houses, gravesites, houses of the recently deceased, ravines, rock outcroppings, and gorges. They said that *mal* is naturally drawn to and gathers at these places, or that it is emitted by spirit beings that occupy these places. Upon contact *mal* sticks (*pega*) to a person and over a short period of time it penetrates and pollutes the entire body. Several informants said *mal* pollution results in internal decay (*decaimiento*). If left untreated the illness is fatal. Children, notably unbaptized children, older adults, and physically debilitated persons are most vulnerable to *mal*.

A constellation of symptoms are associated with *mal aire/mal viento*, manifesting in various combinations of coldness, diarrhea, headache, vomiting, paleness, fatigue, and shaking.

Espanto/Susto

Like *mal aire/mal viento*, *espanto/susto* is a folk illness recognized in other parts of Latin America and among Latino populations in the United States. Generally defined as magical fright, some investigations in the highlands report that *espanto* and *susto* are different illnesses, the former defined as soul loss caused by a frightening experience and the latter as milder form fright sickness. Most of the curanderos interviewed for this investigation, however, agreed that the two terms are synonomous and refer to an illness caused by a frightening experience that, if severe, results in soul loss. Infants and children are particularly susceptible. Some examples of causation shared by informants were an unexpected encounter with a wild animal, an uncommonly aggressive domestic animal, or a spirit being; scary dreams; an accident such as falling down, a car wreck, and a mishap with a tool; and a near accident such as almost being hit by a car or drowning. Receiving distressing news such as the death of a loved one was also reported. Informants explained that the departure of the soul is a dangerous circumstance because *mal* is attracted to and suffuses a souless body. Thus, as with *mal aire/mal viento*, a *limpieza* must be performed to clean the body of *mal* pollution. Symptoms of *espanto/susto* mentioned by informants varied but those most frequently mentioned were loss of appetite, vomiting, crying, sunken eyes, stomach ache, insomnia, and bad dreams.

Mal prójimo, duende, and brujería

Other less frequently mentioned folk illnesses involving magical plant therapy mentioned in the interviews were *mal prójimo*, *duende*, and *brujería*. As described by informants and other investigators, *mal prójimo* ("evil or bad neighbor") is an illness caused by the negative thoughts and feelings that a person or group of people has or have for another individual. The negative thoughts and feelings manifest as a destructive force or energy, described by some informants as *vibraciones* (vibrations) that harm the target individual. It is dynamically similar to another folk illness identified in the highlands known as *envidia* ("envy"). *Duende* ("spirit") is an illness caused by an encounter with a spirit being that dwells in the countryside. *Brujería* (witchcraft) was mentioned by informants in the context of *brujos* (witches) manipulating negative energy to cause harm to others.

La Limpieza

Etiologically, all the folk illnesses discussed above are conceptually linked to *mal* pollution. The function of the *limpieza* is to restore good health by cleansing *mal* from the body. The focus of this paper is the use of magical plants in the *limpieza* for *mal* removal, but it should be noted that informants mentioned a variety of non-plant materia medica used for the same purpose. These materials have been noted in other reports on the *limpieza* in the highlands as well as other parts of Latin America. The non-plant materials most frequently mentioned by informants include eggs, guinea pigs, *trago* (a sugar cane liquor, also known as *aguardiente*), holy water, candles, cologne, chickens, a sweaty shirt, and an over-the-counter bottled essence purchased at markets, "Seven Spirits." Some informants employ idiosyncratic power objects: a dog's skull, a doll's head, and dove's blood. As noted in other sources, the informants use eggs and guinea pigs for both diagnosing and curing folk illnesses. More often than not, the curanderos resort to a combination of plant and non-plant materials for the *limpezia.* The variety of combinations reported by the informants defies description.

A *limpieza* is performed when needed, but some informants indicated that it is most effective if done on a Tuesday or Friday between 6:00 p.m. and midnight. Depending on the degree of *mal* pollution, a *limpieza* may require several sessions. Curanderos first assess the physical symptoms and perform a diagnosis. Typically, a patient is asked to strip down to his underwear and a guinea pig or an egg is rubbed all over his body. Following the rubbing, the guinea pig, described by some informants as functioning like a *radiografía* (x-ray), is slit open ventrally while still alive and then splayed apart. The heart, liver, stomach, intestines, and lungs are examined. The extent of discoloration or disfiguration of the organs indicates the kind of illness. Eggs are cracked open in a glass of water and examined in terms of buoyancy in the water, coloration, and configuration. Others blow cigarette smoke on the arms and legs and observe whether the smoke adheres closely to the skin. If it does, then *mal* pollution is evident.

MAGICAL PLANT CHARACTERISTICS AND USES

It appears that the primary shared characteristic of the plants listed in Table below is odoriferousness. As explained by the informants, it is the scent of leaves or flowers of plants like chilca (*Baccharis obtusifolia*), pumin (*Minthostachys mollis*), clavel (*Dianthus caryophylis*), eucalipto (*Eucalyptus globulus*), marco (*Ambrosia arborecens*), capulí (*Prunus serotina*), hierba buena (*Mentha* × *piperita*), Santa María (*Tanacetum parthenium*), romero (*Rosmarinus officinalis*), and ruda (*Ruta graveolens*) that attracts and draws *mal* from within the body to the surface of the skin and into the plant. Though less frequently mentioned, the fruit or rind of limón (*Citrus medica*) is also used because of its strong odor. More often than not, these plants are used topically. The most common method is to take branches of one or more plants and weave them together to form a whisk broom variously called an *escobita* or *ramos benditos* (holy branches). Some curanderos warm the broom over a fire to pull out a plant's scent. The patient is then brushed with the broom from head to foot.

Other methods of topical administration were reported. Some curanderos rub the leaves of plants together in their hands or crush them in a bowl to enhance the scent and then rub their scented hands or the crushed plants on the patient. Others said that they make a decoction of the plants by boiling them in a pot and then spraying the decoction on the patient by mouth or with a tube. A related method involves placing the patient on a mat, sitting or standing, and pouring or spraying the decoction on him and then rubbing the decoction into the skin. A few informants reported immersing the patient in a bath of clavel flowers. Infusions are also employed, ostensibly for forcing *mal* out of the body. Plants used as infusions include the aforementioned hierba buena, romero, and marco, but also valeriana (*Valeriana decussata*). Having the patient inhale vapors from a hot decoction of eucalipto leaves was mentioned by some informants as another method for forcing *mal* out of the body. As noted earlier, tobacco smoke (*Nicotiana tabacum*) from a cigarette is used for diagnosis, but it is also thought to be effective for pulling *mal* out of the body. Smoke is blown all over a patient's body. The notion of something odorous drawing *mal* from the body is evident in other materia medica used in a *limpieza* such as cologne and the over-the-counter popular magic product mentioned earlier, "Seven Spirits," both of which are sprayed by mouth on the patient's body. It is also illustrated in one curandero's use of a sweaty shirt. He told a story of a client who said that he had been unexpectedly hit by a *huracán* (dust devil or twister) while working in a field. The informant and the client agreed that the *huracán* was the manifestation of a spirit and that the client was polluted with *mal*. Treatment entailed the curandero running about his farm until he produced a sweat soaked shirt smelling strongly of body odor which he used to rub down his client's body.

Informants were not asked if the magical plants used in the *limpieza* are *caliente* (hot), *fresca* (cold) or *templada* (neither hot nor cold), but according to Kothari's and Lombeyda's research on medicinal plants in the highlands (the Imbabura and Bolivar Provinces, respectively), 10 (58.8%) of the 17 plants listed in Table below are *caliente*, two are *fresca*, one is *templada*, and four are not classified. Further research might identify a humoral determinant in the selection of plants for treating folk illnesses.

Magical plants are not only used for cleaning people of *mal* pollution, but also for the *sahumerio*, a ritual used to remove *mal* from a house. Informants said that a *sahumerio* is performed when a family moves into a house that has been abandoned for a lengthy period of time, when someone has died in the house, and when a family has experienced an abnormal number of misfortunes like crop failure, death of livestock, death of relative, loss of employment, and accidents. The house is cleaned by burning incense and/or sweeping the floors, walls, and ceilings of a house with plants like Santa Maria, marco, chilca, and ruda.

The plants used in a *limpieza* are gathered in the wild, purchased in local markets, or, as observed by Finnerman and Sackett, some (e.g., clavel, hierba buena., romero, and ruda) are cultivated in *huertas* (home gardens). It should be noted that, though curanderos are considered more capable of performing a *limpieza* because they have *el don* (the gift) or *el mano bueno* (the good hand), lay people also perform the *limpieza* at home, especially for children.

Following a *limpezia*, the plants and other materials used for cleaning are carefully disposed since they contain harmful *mal* and are viewed much like radioactive and medical waste. One must dispose of them in a place far removed from human habitation and concourse to prevent *mal* contagion of others. As observed by McKee, *mal* cannot be destroyed; it is gradually released back into nature from the healing materials that temporarily contained it.

CONCLUSION

The treatment of folk illnesses constitutes the major part of the practices of the curanderos interviewed by this investigation. All of them reported that they perform the *limpieza* for the treatment of *espanto/susto, mal aire/mal viento, mal prójimo, duende*, and *brujería*. Physicians are not capable of diagnosing and treating these illnesses; only a *limpiador* can.

Of the magical plants reported, only one, guanto rojo (*Datura sanguinea*), belongs to the hallucinogenic category of magical plants, but it is not ingested. Notably absent among the hallucinogenic magical plants indigenous to the highlands is San Pedro cactus (*Echinopsis pachanoi*), an integral element of the culturally similar Quechua ethnomedical tradition in northern Peru. This plant can be gathered in some parts of the Ecuador highlands or purchased in some of the local markets. Recent research on medicinal plants in the Loja Province in the southern portion of the highlands by

Bussman and Sharon noted the absence of its use among curanderos there. They speculate that it was likely used in the past but was abandoned due to its prohibition by the government and church, but we know of no evidence of the use of San Pedro in the highlands during or prior to the conquest period. Other hallucinogenic magical plants not mentioned by the informants include several species indigenous to the Oriente (rainforest) section of Ecuador such as *Banisteriopsis caapi* and *Psychotria viridis*. In conversations with residents of the highlands, several said that the Oriente has many plants with *más poder* (more power), referring to the plants' hallucinogenic properties. According to Saloman, the visionary and curing tradition of the shamans in the Oriente has been held in awe by the highlands residents for hundreds of years. Some of the hallucinogenic plants from the Oriente are available in local markets in the highlands and through traveling herb dealers that make a yearly circuit encompassing the highlands and the Oriente, but none of the curanderos interviewed for this study employ them. This absence is perhaps attributable to no shamans being interviewed for this investigation.

Understood within the context of their use, magical plants reveal the central, single-most important integrative concept of the supernatural component of *curanderismo* in the Ecuador highlands: *el mal*. (Note again that many of the residents interviewed by this study did not use this term. Other terms used to identify the same concept include "energy," "power," and "force." Following McKee, we elected to use the term *mal*.) The concept is directly connected to the etiology and treatment of a wide array of folk illnesses, not only in the Ecuador highlands but also in other parts of Central and South America. It is unclear if the concept of *el mal* is derived from Spanish or indigenous sources, but it is apparent that both mestizo and indigenous residents of the highlands believe in *el mal* and the efficacy of the *limpieza*. In her study of ethnomedicine in Guaranda, a predominantly mestizo town in the highlands, Lombeyda observes that many of the better educated mestizos publically dismiss curanderos as ignorant illiterates and witches while at the same time secretly using their services. We know several mestizos as well as some who claim a blanco identity, including physicians, who frequently seek the help of curanderos for a *limpieza* and other services. On another level, the *mal* concept provides a portal into the mindscape of some highlanders, i.e., the symbolic transmutation of the physical features of the landscape into places that are topophobically perceived as charged with dangerous animate and inanimate forces. These places are akin to what cultural geographers call "landscapes of fear", "sick places", or "landscapes of despair". This topophobic aspect has been identified among other mestizo and indigenous populations in the Ecuador highlands, Bolivia, and Peru. It is a mindscape deeply rooted in what historian MacCormack calls the "sacred topography" of the pre-Christian, Incan, and pre-Incan era, a time when "the plains and the mountains, the sky and the waters were both the theatre and the dramatis personae of divine action (p.146)." She notes that for many contemporary Andeans, "earth and sky are still inhabited by the ancient powers" [p. 433]. As noted by anthropologist George Foster, the highlanders' mindscape was also influenced by beliefs from Spain concerning dangerous "airs" emitted from gravesites and evil spirits riding the wind.

We do not intend to impart the notion that the residents of the highlands live in a constant state of fear of malevolent forces; rather, it is recognition of a living landscape that the highlanders must carefully navigate and negotiate. Conversely, there are therapeutic landscapes in the highlands, places symbolically associated with health and healing such as cathedrals, shrines, lakes, and waterfalls. Furthermore, there is the countervailing and overarching Quichua (or in Peru, Quichua) concept of *pacha mama*, the vital force of "mother nature" that suffuses and sustains all living things. For Catholic highlanders, God does the same. Thus, it is the vital, benevolent power of *pacha mama* or God that flows through the magical plants used by humans to defend themselves against the debilitating and sometimes fatal effect of *mal*.

17

Ethnopharmacological Survey of Six Medicinal Plants

An ethnopharmacological survey was carried out to collect information about the use of six medicinal plants in the regions around Siby and Dioila, Mali. The plants investigated were *Biopyhtum petersianum, Cola cordifolia, Combretum molle, Opilia celtidifolia, Parkia biglobosa* and *Ximenia americana.*

More than 60 medical indications were reported for the use of these plants in traditional medicine. The most frequently reported ailments were malaria (25.6%), different types of pain (14.0%) and dermatitis (7.4%). The main forms for preparation were decoction (58.1%) and powdered plant material (28.4%). The most frequent used plant parts were leaves (37.7%) and stem bark (18.6%). The healers' consensus for the main indications is fairly high for the four plants *B. petersianum, C. cordifolia, C. molle* and *O. celtidifolia*, and this supports the traditional use of these plants. However for *P. biglobosa* and *X. americana* the healers' consensus is less consistent and it is more difficult to draw conclusions about the most important traditional use of these two plants.

BACKGROUND

Mali is a landlocked country located in West-Africa, with an area of approximately 1,246,000 km^2 for an estimated 13.5 million inhabitants. The country is composed of various climatic zones and a diversity of ethnic groups. The life expectancy in Mali is about 44 years for males and 47 years for females. This disturbing health situation of short life expectancy is due to the predominance of infectious diseases and parasites. To improve their health, people use both conventional and traditional medicine. In 2004 the density of physicians in Mali was 0.08 per 1000 inhabitants while already in 1978 there was one healer per 500 inhabitants in Mali.

Traditional medicine still remains the main resource for a large majority of people treating health problems. Being a comprehensive knowledge system, traditional medicine encompasses the utilization of substances, dosages and practices based on socio-cultural norms and religious beliefs as well as witnessed experiences and observations of a specific group. This knowledge is handed down from generation to generation in order to diagnose, prevent or eliminate a physical, social or spiritual imbalance.

In Mali, the Department of Traditional Medicine (DMT) is a collaborating centre of the World Health Organization (WHO) research for traditional medicine. The DMT has as one of their primary objectives to assure that traditional medicine is complementary to conventional medicine, assuming that the medicines can be produced from local resources, especially from medicinal plants. DMT has carried out many phytochemical, pharmacological and toxicological studies with the ultimate goal of providing effective and non-toxic medicine to the population. There are several factors that are taken into account when selecting plants to be studied. One important factor is that several healers from different regions use the same plant to treat the same disease, and that the disease which the plant is used against represents a public health problem. From this work seven improved traditional medicines (ITMs) have been recognized as essential medicines in Mali and are being sold alongside conventional medicines in pharmacies.

The plants in our survey were chosen by DMT as they want to investigate if these plants are suitable candidates for development into new ITMs.

METHODOLOGY

An ethnopharmacological survey was carried out in the regions around Siby and Dioila in November and December 2007, and a total of 58 healers were interviewed. 27 healers in the villages Siby, Dogoro and Gouena (Siby area) and 1 healer in the village Sirimabougou (Dioila area) were interviewed about the medicinal usage of *Biophytum petersianum* Klotzsch. (Oxalidaceae) and *Opilia celtidifolia* Endl. ex Walp. (Opiliaceae). 30 healers in the villages Banko, Sirimabougou and Ngolobougou (Dioila area) were interviewed about the medicinal usage of *Cola cordifolia* Sim (Sterculiaceae), *Combretum molle* R.Br. ex G.Don. (Combretaceae), *Parkia biglobosa* Benth. (Leguminosae) and *Ximenia americana* L. (Olacaceae).

The healers were asked whether or not they were using the plants in their practice. When a healer was using a plant in his practice, the information collected also included indication, part(s) of the plant being used, method(s) of preparation and details of administration, including the approximate amounts and number of doses per day.

In some cases the healers reported the use of the *Loranthus spp.* when asked about a specific plant.

Although the *Loranthus spp.* is distinct species it is discussed as a part of the plant it grows on because the healers see it as a part of the plant in question. The interviews were performed in the Bambara language with Professor Drissa Diallo and Doctor Sekou Bah, DMT, Bamako, and Ngolo Ballo, a plant systematist at DMT, as interpreters.

Prior to the interviews the healers were given information about the project, the participants in the survey and its goals. In respect of tradition, gifts of cola nuts (*Cola nitida* (Sterculiaceae)) and money were bestowed upon the traditional healers. The conversations with the healers are built on trust with the common goal of increasing the knowledge on medicinal plants and improving the health situation in the country.

RESULTS AND DISCUSSION

Biophytum petersianum *Klotzsch. (Oxalidaceae)*

= *Biophytum sensitivum* (L.) DC. (Oxalidaceae) and *Oxalis sensitiva* L. (Oxalidaceae)

LOCAL NAME: YELENI NÈLOUTOGO AND DJUTOGOUI

Biopyhtum petersianum is a slender annual herb with stems up to 25 cm long; it has leaves in a terminal crown which are very sensitive. It is widespread in tropical and subtropical Africa, and across Asia to New Guinea.

Traditional Use

For *B. petersianum* the main indication in our survey was cerebral malaria (58.1% of the reported ailments for *B. petersianum*), while treatment of different types of pain was the second most cited ailment (9.7%). Various other ailments were also reported. A preparation of a powder from the plant was the most common preparation (41.9%) followed by a combination of powder and decoction (32.3%) and decoction (19.4%). The whole plant is the most frequent plant part used. The healers' agreement about the main indication is fairly high and this supports the traditional use of *B. petersianum* against cerebral malaria.

BIOLOGICAL ACTIVITIES

Methanolic extract has shown effect on COX-2 expression, and different types of polyphenolic compounds, some with effect on the COX-1/-2 system, have been isolated from *B.* sensitivum. Different types of extracts from the plant have shown anti-inflammatory activity on the carrageenan-rat paw endema and complement fixing polysaccharides from the plant have been reported. The results above may explain the traditional use in treatment of malaria as the complement system is a part of the innate immune system and activating of the immune system can accelerate the body's immune response to malaria. The use in treatment of pain may be explained by the plant extract's modulation of COX expression and anti-inflammatory activity. Guruvayoorappan and Kuttan have recently been performing a large scale investigation of antitumor effects of *Biophytum sensitivum*, and they have found that methanolic extracts of *B. sensitivum* have apoptotic effect on B16F-10 cells, and regulatory effects on NO- and cytokine production on tumor-associated macrophages. They also found that the methanolic extract stimulates the immune cell system in mice, leading to immune cell proliferation and that this, in turn, can stimulate NK cell-mediated tumor lysis.

COLA CORDIFOLIA *SIM (STERCULIACEAE)*

Local Name: N'tabanokò

Cola cordifolia grows on the savannah in Senegal to Mali and is a large tree up to 15–25 m high, with a short buttressed trunk, low-branching with a dense crown.

Traditional Use

Cola cordifolia is a remedy used to cure several diseases. In our survey different types of pain is the most frequent reported ailment (35.1% of the reported ailments for *C. cordifolia*) followed by fever (13.5%) and diarrhoea (10.8%). Various other ailments were also reported. The stem bark of *C. cordifolia* was used most frequently (51.4%) followed by the *Loranthus spp.* of the plant (13.5%) and the combination of leaves and stem bark (10.8%). The two most used preparations were decoction (67.6%) and preparation of a powder (24.3%). The decoction is usually used for a bath and/or to drink. The powder is usually dissolved in water and used for a bath and/or to drink, or the powder is thrown into fire and the smoke is inhaled. The healers' consensus for the main indication is fairly high, and this supports the traditional use of *C. cordifolia* as a remedy to treat different types of pain.

According to literature a decoction of the powdered bark of *C. cordifolia* is used in Mali for treatment of old wounds. An ethnopharmacological survey carried out in the areas around Dioila and Bandiagara, Mali, indicated that the plant was used in treating a wide variety of ailments. The bark is also used in Casamance, Senegal, in maceration for chest-affections, and together with other medicinal plants for blennorrhoea. A water-concoction is drunk in The Gambia for constipation, and the inner bark applied to a swollen finger is said to hasten maturation of pus.

Maceration of the twigs is administered in Casamance, Senegal, to facilitate childbirth. Water in which split-up small branches have been soaked is taken in The Gambia as a diuretic. A leaf-macerate is used in Senegal in leprosy treatment, and sap from leaf petioles is used in The Gambia in eye-treatments.

Root taken from the eastside of the tree, split up and put in a bottle with water is deemed helpful in The Gambia to get rid of gonorrhoea.

Biological Activities

Despite the traditional medicinal use of the plant, few studies have been performed on the plant. In 1988 Diop et al. investigated the Vitamin C content in fresh fruits from West-Africa. Togola et al. found that the crude water extract had complement fixing activity and this could implement a role in activating the immune system. These results may explain the medicinal use since the activating of the immune system is involved in the immune response fighting diseases.

COMBRETUM MOLLE *R.BR. EX G.DON. (COMBRETACEAE)*

Local Name: Ganianka

Combretum molle is a shrub or small tree to 10 m high, rarely 16 m, with a straight regular bole to 1 m girth, of savannah forest, from Senegal to West-Cameroon, and widespread in tropical Africa.

Traditional Use

Combretum molle is used as a remedy to cure several diseases. In our survey the main indication is malaria (62.5% of the reported ailments for *C. molle*) followed by different types of pain (12.5%).

Various other ailments were also reported. The most frequent part of the plant used is the leaves (75.0%) and the *Loranthus spp.* of the plant (15.0%). Decoction (80.0%) and a preparation of powder (17.5%) are the most commonly used preparations. The decoction is usually used for a bath and/or to drink. The powder is usually suspended in water and used for a bath and/or to drink, or the powder is thrown into fire and the smoke is inhaled. The healers' agreement about the main indication is fairly high and this supports the traditional use of *C. molle* against malaria.

4 healers used the *Loranthus spp.* of *C. molle* for fortune seeking and to chase away evil spirits/and curses.

According to the literature *C. molle* is used in wound healing procedures in the Bamako region, Mali. In Senegal the plant is held to be cholagogic, but inferior to *Combretum crotonoides* (Combretaceae) and *Combretum micranthum* (Combretaceae), and an aqueous suspension of powdered bark together with the mumuye gum is used as a gargle and in draught for sore-throat. The Dagarar of Burkina Faso applies powdered bark to sores. The bark along with cereal foods is taken for dysentery, and is used in ceremonial preparation for young children to prevent sickness and other troubles.

Leaves are prepared as a decoction for baths and draughts, or powdered and added to food in treatment of dropsy, ascites and oedemas in Senegal. In Ivory Coast and Nigeria this plant is used in the absence of that popular panacea, kinkeliba (*C. micranthum*) for treating jaundice and yellow fever, and in Burkina Faso it is given for abdominal complaints, diarrhoea etc., blennorrhoea, anuria, etc., and sometimes to women in childbirth to hasten the expulsion of the after-birth.

Lobi of Burkina Faso often takes a decoction of leafy twigs in draughts and baths for bronchial affections and Bobo of Ivory Coast consider the plant a poison-antidote. The Maninka also treats whitlows by steeping the affected part in a leaf-decoction. Alcoholic extracts of leaves with water extracts of twigs have shown capacity to reduce sarcoma tumors in animals.

In the southern part of Senegal the plant is ascribed with magical properties by the Fula and Fouladou to promote courage in battle by inhaling smoke emitted from fire on which bark and branches have been placed. The wood is never used to stoke domestic hearths.

Biological Activities

Some studies have been performed on the biological activities of *C. molle*. Ojewole found analgesic, anti-inflammatory and cardiovascular effects of mollic acid glucoside isolated from *C. molle* leaves. Asres et al. reported that the acetone extract of leaves from *C. molle* has antiprotozoal activity. In an investigation of the biological activity of different *Combretum spp.* McGaw et al. found *C. molle* to have both anti-inflammatory and antischistosomal activity. These findings indicating that *C. molle* has antiprotozoal and anti-inflammatory activity may explain the traditional use of the plant against malaria and pain.

OPILIA CELTIDIFOLIA *ENDL. EX WALP.* *(OPILIACEAE)*

Local Name: Korôgué

Opilia celtidifolia is a woody climber, spreading, heavily-branched shrub or tree up to 10 m high, which grows in fringing forest and savannah, often on anthills. It is widespread from Senegal to Nigeria and dispersed over the drier parts of tropical Africa.

Traditional Use

The main indication for *O. celtidifolia* in our survey was dermatitis (51.6% of the reported ailments for *O. celtidifolia*). The use of *O. celtidifolia* in treatment of dermatitis in Mali has also been previously reported by Togola et al. in 2005, where an ethnopharmacological survey showed that dermatitis was the main indication. In Mali the term dermatitis is used as a common term for all kinds of skin disorders. Various other ailments were also reported, but only one or two healers reported usage of the plant for each ailment. The leaves of *O. celtidifolia* are the most frequent plant part used in traditional medicine (87.1% of the cases), and a decoction (64.5%) is the most common preparation. The healers' consensus for the main indication is fairly high, and this supports the traditional use of *O. celtidifolia* as a remedy to treat dermatitis.

According to the literature the leaves of *O. celtidifolia* are mainly used to treat dermatitis and malaria in Mali, but the plant is also used in wound healing procedures. A decoction of the leaves is used against fever in Ivory Coast.

In Senegal a decoction is used as a gargle for dental abscesses, to treat oedema and as a general stimulant. The plant has internal and external use; against leprosy, acting as a purgative, and leaves reduced to ash are used against headache. The plant is said to have a violent action on the digestion system, and the stem and root are anthelmintic. In Nigeria the plant is primarily used in veterinary medicine.

Biological activities

In the literature there are only a few surveys on the biological activity of *O. celtidifolia*, most of the previous work have been focused on the chemistry of the plant. Togola et al. isolated polysaccharides with complement fixing and macrophage stimulating activity from the water extract. Both the complement system and the macrophages are part of the immune system and play a role in the wound healing process.

The activation of these processes may indicate that the polysaccharides from *O. celtidifolia* play a role in the wound healing process and this could explain the extensive use of different leaf preparations against dermatitis in Mali. In earlier work Shihata et al. isolated saponins from the methanol extract and found anthelmintic and antispasmodic activities for these compounds. Saponins are reported to have a number of biological activities, among them immunostimulatory, antipyretic and antiparasitic effects. The effects shown for saponins could explain the use of *O. celtidifolia* as a remedy for dermatitis, fever and internal worms.

PARKIA BIGLOBOSA *BENTH. (LEGUMINOSAE)*

Local Name: Nèrè

Parkia biglobosa is a tree being up to 20 m high, bole stout, not butteressed, low-branching, bearing a large wide-spreading crown, deciduous, flowering while leafless; flowers in pendulous capitula bearing also pendulous, large fruit pods; of the Soudanian/Guinean savannah and transition woodland, from Senegal across the Region and on into southern Sudan.

Traditional Use

Parkia biglobosa is used as a remedy in our survey to treat different types of wounds (16.2% of the reported ailments for *P. biglobosa*) and pain (10.8%), and these are the most frequent reported ailments followed fungal infection (8.1%). *Parkia biglobosa* is also used against various other ailments. The stem bark of *P. biglobosa* was used most frequently (56.8%) followed by the leaves of the plant (21.6%). The two most used preparations were decoction (62.2%) and preparation of a powder (29.7%).

The decoction is usually used for a bath and/or to drink. The powder is usually dissolved in water and used for a bath and/or to drink, or the powder is thrown into fire and the smoke is inhaled. The healers' agreement for the main indication for *P. biglobosa* is relatively low and it is therefore more difficult to pinpoint the most important traditional use of this plant.

2 healers used *P. biglobosa* for fortune seeking and to chase away evil spirits/and curses.

According to the literature the leaves, bark and pods are used to treat new and old wounds in Dogonland, Mali. The bark-infusion is taken in Kordofanan in Ivory Coast, Burkina Faso and South-East Nigeria as a tonic and anti-diarrhoetic. The bark is commonly sold in herbalist shops in the western part of the Region for the analgesic action it confers in mouthwashes and steam-inhalations for toothache. A red colour is imparted to the mouth while the saponins in the bark contribute asepsis. In Casmance, Senegal, the bark has wide usage: alone for female sterility, baths and by draughts, and similarly administrated in prescription with other drug-plants for skin-infections and leprosy, and for blennorrhoea.

Fula and Tukulor people of Senegal drink a decoction against *Schistosoma* infection. In Ivory Coast and Burkina Faso the pounded bark with lemon juice added is applied to sores and ulcers; a decoction is considered anti-rachitic, tonic and febrifugal; and it is one of 32 other plants in a complex prescription used in the Kaya region for leprosy. The bark is chewed by men in The Gambia for lack of virility; the cause will then, it is said, be voided on going to the latrine.

The leaves have some undefined medicinal use in Niger. In Nigeria and The Gambia root and leaf are pounded together in water to produce an eye-lotion. In Senegal medicinal use of the leaf is restricted to external applications. The leaves (and bark) are used in eye-lotion.

The crushed leaf is made up into poultices, and to dab on the lips to dissipate 'fever spots'. They are made into steam inhalations in The Gambia for toothache. Lightly heated, then crushed, the leaflets are applied to burns.

Biological Activities

Agunu et al. reported that *P. biglobosa* showed anti-diarrhoeal properties in mice. Kouadio et al. showed that the hexane extract from the bark of *P. biglobosa* had some analgesic and anti-inflammatory effects. Asuzu and Harvey reported the methanol extract of *P. biglobosa* has shown significant protection against the neurotoxic, haemotoxic and cytotoxic effects of venoms of poisonous snakes. Studies have been done to identify the chemical constituents of the bark, Araujo et al. found sterols and triterpenes in the petroleum ether extract and Tringali et al. identified long-chain ester of *trans*-ferulic acid, a mixture of long-chain *cis*-ferulates and different kinds of catechins. Catechins and ferulates are antioxidants, and their antioxidant properties may be responsible for some of the medicinal effect seen for this plant.

XIMENIA AMERICANA *L. (OLACACEAE)*

Local Name: Ntonkè

Ximenia americana is a very variable shrubby tree up to 5 m high. It is often semi-parasitic, with strong thorns, or thornless, in savannah. The tree grows from Senegal to West Cameroon and is also widely dispersed in tropical Africa, America and Asia.

Traditional Use

Ximenia americana is used as a remedy to cure several diseases. In our survey throat infection (12.8% of the reported ailments for *X. americana*) and malaria (12.8%) are the most frequent reported ailments followed by dysmenorrhoea (10.3%). The roots (48.7%) and leaves (30.8%) are most frequently used in the treatment of the ailments. The two most used preparations were decoction (48.7%) and preparation of a powder (43.6%). The decoction is usually used for a bath and/or to drink. The powder is usually dispersed in water and used for a bath and/or to drink, or the powder is thrown into fire and the smoke is inhaled. The healers' consensus is less consistent for *X. americana* and it is therefore more difficult to say which medical indication that is the most important one.

4 healers used the *Loranthus spp.* of *X. americana* for fortune seeking and to chase away evil spirits/and curses.

According to the literature *X. americana* is well known for its medicinal properties, and all parts of the tree are used. In Mali wounds are treated with a wash with a decoction of leaves or a combination of a wash with a decoction of bark and applying powdered bark is to the wounds. Powder from bark is used on insect stings leading to boils. The pulverised bark and roots are used in West Africa on epidermal troubles: on ulcers, craw-craw, ringworm, sores, etc. Powdered bark is deemed to be a good cleansing agent. Tenda in Casamance, Senegal, soak infected feet in boiled water with crushed bark and salt and bind them in cloth overnight, and then dead skin will be sloughed off. Root-bark is put into febrifugal medicines in Casamance, Senegal, and the plant is used against schistosomiasis in Ivory Coast, Burkina Faso and Nigeria. The roots have internal uses in Casamance, Senegal, to treat guinea-worm infection, against leprosy and impotence, and in Nigeria for fever diarrhoea, jaundice, stomatitis and toothache. For swelling of the face, powdered root is inhaled in Senegal in mixture with *Maerua angolensis* (Capparaceae). In Tanganyika, Ivory Coast and Burkina Faso the root is used against fevers and diarrhoea. Root-powder massaged on the gums is used in Ivory Coast and Burkina Faso for stomatitis and toothache. The root compounded with the root of *Annona chrysophylla* (Annonaceae) has been used in Nigeria for sleeping-sickness.

Biological Activities

Voss et al. found the water extract of *X. americana* to have potent anticancer activity and that this effect was due to a type II ribosome-inactivating protein, riproximin. Asres et al. reported that extract from the stem bark of *X. americana* had antiviral activity against human immunodeficiency virus type 1 (HIV-1) and type 2 (HIV-2). Kone et. al found that extract of *X. americana* to have antibacterial effect. Omer and Elnima tested extracts of different polarity and from different parts of the plant and found the methanolic and aqueous extracts to have antimicrobial effects. Diallo et al. reported that water extract from *X. americana* have a complement fixing ability. The results showing that *X. americana* have complement fixing and antimicrobial effect could explain the plants traditional use against infections and malaria in Mali.

PLANT PARTS USED AND MODE OF PREPARATION

Overall in our survey the leaves are the most frequently used plant part (37.7% of the citations for all plants), followed by the stem bark, the whole plant and the roots, 18.6%, 13.0% and 10.7% respectively. Preparations made of other plant parts and combinations of the parts mention above are more unusual, ranging from 0.5 – 2.8%. The usages of the *Loranthus spp.* growing on the different medicinal plants were also reported quite frequently (6.5%) compared to earlier ethnopharmacological studies performed in Mali (usage not reported and unpublished results).

In another ethnopharmacological study of medicinal plants in Dioila, Kolokani and Siby (Mali), Togola et al. reported that the leaves (56.3%) and the roots (30.0%) were the most frequently used plant parts. The leaves (22%) and the roots (24%) were also the most frequently used parts in a survey performed in Dogonland (Mali) by Inngjerdingen et al. in 2004. That the leaves are the most frequently used plant parts corresponds well with our own findings, but we found the stem bark to be the second most cited plant part used. The roots was only used 10.7% of the cases. There could be many reasons for this, but one explanation could be that the different surveys have been focused on different medicinal plants.

In our survey the overall results for used plant parts differ from the results of *C. cordifolia*, *P. biglobosa* and *X. americana*. The stem bark was the most frequent used plant part of *C. cordifolia* (51.4%) and *P. biglobosa* (56.8%). For *X. americana* the most frequent plant part used is the root (48.7%). Togola et al. reported that the need and use of stem bark increased during the dry and windy season from February to May due to the lack of leaves during this period. Our survey was carried out in November-December after the rainy season so lack of leaves is probably not the explanation for the use of stem bark and roots in this case. A number of the healers also told us that they used stem bark from different sides of the tree (North, East, South and West). The reason for this could be to ensure that the tree will survive when they are collecting the bark, because removing larger areas of bark from just one side of the tree could expose so much of the trunk that the tree might acquire diseases and eventually dies.

Decoction was by far the most used method of preparation (58.1% of the citations for all plants) followed by powder and a combination of decoction and powder (28.4% and 7.0% respectively). Other methods of preparations were also used, but only to a minor extent. In another study performed by Togola et al. decoction was also the most frequent way of preparation (65%) followed by infusion of powder (13%). These findings are similar to the results of our study.

ADMINISTRATION AND DOSAGE

Oral and external applications as wash, steam bath or ointment are the administration forms that are most frequently used. Inhalation of steam was used in treatment of throat infections and fumigation was often used in the treatment of headache.

Different types of additives are sometimes used by the healers when preparing the remedies. Salt, food and drinks are used to improve taste of the preparation and thus the patients' compliance. Butter, oil and mud are used to make ointments or liniments for external use of the medicinal plants. The healers in our survey in some cases also used the combination of different medicinal plants to treat ailments.

For most ailments and remedies, the dosage given depends upon the sex, age, duration of illness, health and physical condition of the patient. The doses vary from 1 teacup for 1 day to 3–4 teacups 3 times a day for several days for oral administration. The same is noted when the treatment is a bath, often it is enough with a bath other times it is required several baths a day for a longer period of time. This variation was also noted when the plant was used to treat the same ailment. Togola et al. suggested that the variation of the doses and duration of treatment from one healer to another may indicate that the plants have a low degree of toxicity. That corresponds well with our survey where the only side effects reported were diarrhoea and vomiting, and only in connection with *O. celtidifolia.*

CONCLUSION

In the present study over 60 medicinal indications were reported for the six medicinal plants investigated. The healers' consensus for the main indications is fairly high for the four plants *B. petersianum, C. cordifolia, C. molle* and *O. celtidifolia*, and this supports the traditional use of these plants. However for *P. biglobosa* and *X. americana* the healers' consensus is less consistent and it is more difficult to draw conclusions about the most important traditional use of these two plants.

This survey complements the ongoing investigation of different medicinal plants from Mali. The ultimate goal for our project is to provide efficient and non-toxic medicines to the population in Mali, where medicinal plants still remains the main resource for a large majority of people treating health problems. Chemical characterization and the biological-, pharmacological- and toxicological activity of the plants are currently under investigation. Plant extract showing bioactivity corresponding to the traditional application of the plant can validate the traditional medicinal usage of the plant. These studies will hopefully provide important knowledge necessary for designing therapeutic agents from the plants.

Bibliography

Farnsworth, N.R.: *Ethnobotany and the search for new drugs (Ciba Foundation Symposium 185)*, Chichester, UK, John Wiley and Sons, 1994.

ITDG & IIRR. *Ethnoveterinary medicine in Kenya: a field manual of traditional animal health care practices.* Nairobi, Intermediate Technology Development Group and International Institute of Rural Reconstruction, 1996.

Martin, P.J.: *Resistance of parasites to antiparasitic drugs.* Rahway. NJ, USA, MSD AGVET, 1990.

McCorkle, C.M.: *Ethnoveterinary Research and Development.* London, Intermediate Technology Publications, 1996.

Minja, M.M.J.: *Proceedings of the 7th Tanzania Veterinary Association Scientific Conference*, Arusha, 1989.

Plotkin, M.J.: *Natural resources and human health: plants of medicinal and nutritional value*, Proceedings, Amsterdam, the Netherlands, Elsevier, 1992.

Roepke, D.A.: *Ethnoveterinary research and development.* London, Intermediate Technology Publications, 1996.

Sofowora, A.: *Medicinal plants and traditional medicine in Africa.* Chichester, UK, John Wiley and Sons, 1982.

Warren, D.M.: *The cultural dimension of development: indigênous knowledge systems.* London, Intermediate Technology Publications, 1995.

Index

□□□